THE
RUNNER'S
DEVOTIONAL

THE
RUNNER'S
DEVOTIONAL

**INSPIRATION AND MOTIVATION FOR LIFE'S JOURNEY...
ON AND OFF THE ROAD**

DANA NIESLUCHOWSKI | DAVE VEERMAN

TYNDALE HOUSE PUBLISHERS, INC.
CAROL STREAM, ILLINOIS

Visit Tyndale online at www.tyndale.com.

TYNDALE and Tyndale's quill logo are registered trademarks of Tyndale House Publishers, Inc.

The Runner's Devotional: Inspiration and Motivation for Life's Journey . . . On and Off the Road

Copyright © 2011 by Livingstone Corporation. All rights reserved.

Cover photograph copyright © John Burcham/National Geographic/Getty. All rights reserved.

Designed by Stephen Vosloo

Edited by Erin Marshall

Unless otherwise indicated, all Scripture quotations are from the *Holy Bible*, New Living Translation, copyright © 1996, 2004, 2007 by Tyndale House Foundation. Used by permission of Tyndale House Publishers, Inc., Carol Stream, Illinois 60188. All rights reserved.

Scripture quotations marked NIV are from the Holy Bible, *New International Version*,® NIV.® Copyright © 1973, 1978, 1984, 2010 by Biblica, Inc.™ Used by permission of Zondervan. All rights reserved worldwide. www.zondervan.com.

"The Runner" for Week 47 is adapted from the "Personality Profile of Barnabas" in the *Life Application Study Bible*, copyright © 1988, 1989, 1990, 1991, 1993, 1996, 2004, 2007 by Tyndale House Publishers, Inc. Used by permission.

"The Runner" for Week 52 is adapted from Meb Keflezighi, *Run to Overcome*, copyright © 2010 by Meb Keflezighi. Used by permission.

Library of Congress Cataloging-in-Publication Data

Niesluchowski, Dana.
   The runner's devotional : inspiration and motivation for life's journey— on and off the road / Dana Niesluchowski and Dave Veerman.
      p. cm.
   Includes bibliographical references (p.   ) and index.
   ISBN 978-1-4143-4812-4 (sc)
1. Runners (Sports)—Prayers and devotions.   2. Running—Religious aspects—Christianity— Prayers and devotions.   I. Veerman, David.   II. Title.
   BV4596.A8N54 2011
   242—dc23   2011020855

Printed in the United States of America

17   16   15   14   13

7   6   5   4   3   2

DEDICATION

To Kara . . .
loving daughter
loyal sister
amazing wife and mother
woman of God.

ABOUT THE AUTHORS

DANA NIESLUCHOWSKI

Dana competed in soccer, swimming, basketball, volleyball, baseball, softball, and more. She loves all sports and is an avid runner, having successfully competed in several races, including a triathlon and a marathon. Dana received her B.S. degree in kinesiology from Wheaton College and her M.A. in exercise physiology from the University of North Carolina, Chapel Hill. At the Livingstone Corporation (a company that partners with Christian publishers to produce Bibles, books, Bible studies, curricula, and other resources), Dana managed and contributed to many resources, including the *Legacy Bible*, *Lose It for Life*, and *iStand—the Power of Courageous Choices*. Recently, she and her dad wrote the *Sports Trivia Devotional*. Dana, her husband, Walter, and young son, Edmund, live in Oswego, Illinois.

DAVE VEERMAN

Dave played high school basketball and football and college football. Since then, he has finished six marathons. A graduate of Wheaton College (B.A.) and Trinity Evangelical Divinity School (M.Div.), Dave has written sixty-five books, including *Parenting Passages*, *How to Apply the Bible*, *Letting Them Go*, *One Year Through the Bible*, and *If I Knew Then What I Know Now*. He also served as a senior editor of the *Life*

Application Study Bible and *Student's Life Application Study Bible*. The father of two athletic daughters (Dana and Kara) and a founding partner of the Livingstone Corporation, Dave and his wife, Gail, live in Naperville, Illinois.

TABLE OF CONTENTS

INTRODUCTION

Runners begin running for a variety of reasons. Many eventually discover that running can be a spiritual experience: a time to pray, observe God's handiwork, think, and learn. Thus, running can serve as an ideal metaphor for spiritual truths. Fittingly, the New Testament includes several references to faith as a race (1 Corinthians 9:24; Galatians 2:2, 5:7; Philippians 2:16, 3:14; 2 Timothy 4:7; Hebrews 12:1).

The purpose of this book is to help anyone, especially runners, deepen their relationship with God. The contents progress from purpose and goals through workouts and then into the race itself—a marathon—with each two weeks highlighting a significant aspect of that journey.

We've written a year's worth of devotionals—fifty-two weeks. And we've divided each week into several sections, all centered on the theme for that week. We've also included a running log for each week. This is a place for you to record time, distance, weather, and notes for five days of runs.

You may want to read one week at one sitting, or you may want to take your time and spend a few days on one devotional. If you would rather keep a daily schedule, here's a suggestion for how to divide each week:

- Monday—Read the narrative at the beginning that introduces the running theme and the Bible passage.

- Tuesday—Read the section titled "The Runner."
- Wednesday—Read these sections: "The Race" and "The Result."
- Thursday—Read "My Story."
- Friday—Answer the questions under "Think It Through."
- Weekend—Take time to fill in the "Journal" page, reflecting back on the week and what you've learned and applied. Read "On Running."

We pray that through this experience you will run in step with your Savior and finish well.

Dana and Dave

THE STARTING LINE

It is the day of the marathon, and what a fantastic group of people has shown up! I give thanks to God for each one and remember Philippians 4:13—"I can do everything through Christ, who gives me strength." I praise God for this glorious opportunity. I have five newbies ready to run 26.2 miles, and they are relying on me to get them to the finish line. I know they really do not need me in order to finish; they just need to be encouraged. I share with them something I always think about, that each runner brings a different story to the starting line and that I have 26.2 miles to learn another runner's story and make new friends along the way.

We are five minutes from the start. . . .

I say, "In five minutes you are going to ask your body to endure 26.2 miles, and each of you has a personal goal and one common goal, to finish your first marathon. Remember that you have put in an incredible amount of training miles and time. Do not lose sight of how you successfully got to the starting line. Run with pride. You will be a different runner when you finish, stronger and wiser to take on any challenges life brings your way. So congratulations, and know I am incredibly proud of you!" We pray together for a great day, an injury-free run, and a happy finish.

Then off we go!

So fun, such amazing energy, and a journey that holds challenges all the way to the finish line. A very good day.

I pray that they will continue to run happily and reflect fondly on all the goals that were achieved during their marathon and the season of training, too. I pray they will remember that what we bring to the starting line or to others at a race is more important than just running our fastest time. We bring a story, joy, encouragement, and a little hope!

Caroline

DETERMINE YOUR PURPOSE

In order to reach your goal at anything in life, you need to know your purpose. Without a purpose, you will lack focus and are destined to run aimlessly. You can go for a run one day, but without having a reason for running (staying fit, losing weight, etc.), the chances are slim that you will continue for more than a couple of days. Your purpose is what will keep you going.

Paul encourages Timothy, his ministry protégé, to remember his purpose—to glorify God and serve Jesus Christ, and in doing this, to be an example to other believers even as a young pastor. In order for Timothy to develop into a good servant, he must grow spiritually, teach others the truths of the gospel message, and model a life of faith and purity. That would be his race.

Train yourself to be godly. "Physical training is good, but training for godliness is much better, promising benefits in this life and in the life to come." This is a trustworthy saying, and everyone should accept it. This is why we work hard

and continue to struggle, for our hope is in the living God,
who is the Savior of all people and particularly of all believers.
(1 TIMOTHY 4:7-10)

The Runner

My doctor's appointment was supposed to be a normal physical exam. I felt great and had no concerns. Sure, I was a little out of shape since my college football days, and my wife had mentioned that I was putting on some weight. But no big deal; I'm just getting old, right?

Then the doctor came in and gave me news that rocked my world and changed my life. "I just did a quick read of your blood results. It shows that you have developed type 2 diabetes," he calmly said.

"What?" I replied. "But I feel great! I'm not tired. . . . Well, I get a little bit winded going up the stairs, but who doesn't? Are you sure?"

"Yep, I'm sure. You are going to have to make some big changes to your lifestyle—starting with exercising, eating better, and losing some weight. Did you know that you have gained twenty pounds since I saw you last year?"

I barely heard the instructions as the nurse told me how to take my blood sugar levels, how to trace them, and what I needed to get started. (Thank goodness she gave me a pamphlet.) I kept thinking, *How can this happen to me? I've always been the athlete and in great shape. What went wrong?* I prayed, *Lord, I don't have to have diabetes, do I? I want to see Darcy and Evan finish high school, graduate from college, get married, and have their own families. And what about Pamela? I need to be there for her. To support her and love her. To help her raise our children.*

I needed to make some changes and fast. So together Pamela and I developed a new eating plan. But the toughest part was starting to exercise. I hadn't tied my laces and stepped out to do any aerobic activity in years. Could I do it? Would I hate it? It didn't matter. I had to get healthy. I knew that running is a good way to lose weight quickly . . . and it is free. I made the decision: I was going to run. The next day

I got up early, put on my shoes, and headed out for my first run since college fifteen years earlier.

The Race

Everyone starts running for a reason. For some it could be a sport that requires them to run a mile at a certain pace. Others receive news from a doctor that underscores their need to exercise. Or maybe a father's new baby girl makes him want to live a healthy life so he can watch her grow up. No matter what your reason, your purpose, at some point you decide to run.

In the same way, as Paul points out, we need to remember our purpose and choose to grow in our faith in God. The message of faith must reach into the heart.

> *Christ will make his home in your hearts as you trust in him.*
> *Your roots will grow down into God's love and keep you strong.*
> *And may you have the power to understand, as all God's*
> *people should, how wide, how long, how high, and how deep*
> *his love is. May you experience the love of Christ, though it is*
> *too great to understand fully. Then you will be made complete*
> *with all the fullness of life and power that comes from God.*
> (EPHESIANS 3:17-19)

Just watching others run won't change your fitness level; you have to do it. In the same way, to become spiritually fit, you must make a decision. And in this way you can "be an example to all believers in what you say, in the way you live, in your love, your faith, and your purity" (1 Timothy 4:12).

The Result

To be a better runner and have more effective workouts, you need to push your body, challenge yourself, and train effectively. But more important than having a good workout is being healthy spiritually—strengthening your relationship with God and persevering in your faith. Do you spend more time focusing on your running routine than on your spiritual practices? Are you using your God-given abilities to minister to others and help them grow in their faith, or do you spend most of your time *thinking* about Christ instead of *being* Christ to those around you?

Remember your spiritual purpose. As you strengthen your legs, increase your breath capacity and develop a good stride for running. Remember that you are also training for godliness in your spiritual race.

My Story

I'm not saying I was drifting through life, but I definitely wasn't living with purpose. In just about every area, I would do what I thought was best for the situation and for me—relationships, career, personal finances, diet, running, and even my faith. And I thought I was doing okay for a twenty-five-year-old. I had plenty of friends and a good job, and I was in good health. But then one Sunday the sermon got me thinking about my purpose for life, why I was on this earth, what I was living for. The pastor preached on 1 Corinthians 10, and highlighting verse 31, he said that the main purpose for all of God's creations should be to glorify him. Paul wrote, "So whether you eat or drink, or whatever you do, do it all for the glory of God."

"*All* for the glory of God"—that includes every aspect of my life. So I asked God to help me do that, and ever since I've tried to remember my purpose. Now at meals, on the job, in the gym, at church, and everywhere else, I consider how I can glorify God through this. I'm not always sure of the answer, but at least I'm asking the right question. Now I live with purpose.

Brian

Think It Through

1. What can someone do to glorify God in a relationship? How about in a marriage and family? What about on the job?
2. How can you, like Timothy, be an "example to all believers"?
3. What's your ultimate purpose for running?
4. What can you do to run "for the glory of God"?

On Running

What are the differences between aerobic and anaerobic activities?

The biggest difference between aerobic and anaerobic activities is how the body supplies energy for the action. Simply put, aerobic = oxygen, and anaerobic = without oxygen; however, it is much more complex than that. Our muscles have a certain amount of ready-to-use carbohydrates in the blood system. Anaerobic activities (weight lifting, activities that take less than one minute, sprints, etc.) quickly use that stored energy. Aerobic activities are longer and require more than just the quick supply in the muscles. Because the body constantly needs energy, more oxygen is needed to create the energy, thus developing the heart and lungs.

JOURNAL

_____

_____

_____

_____

_____

_____

_____

RUNNING LOG

	TIME	DISTANCE	WEATHER	NOTES
DAY 1				
DAY 2				
DAY 3				
DAY 4				
DAY 5				

DETERMINE YOUR PURPOSE

Imagine packing your suitcase, loading the car, and filling your car with gas. Excited for your vacation, you hit the road. But after a few miles, you realize that you have no idea where you are headed. Will you get anywhere? Doubtful. Because you don't have a destination in mind, you will probably just drive in circles.

Often we treat faith the same way. We read the Bible, go to church, and volunteer, but we still feel as if we are just going in circles. Those activities are good and important, but unless we have a good reason for doing them—a desired destination—we won't make much progress in the Christian journey. When giving instructions to his young pastor friend, Paul told Timothy that he needed to run his "race" with purpose: "But you, Timothy, are a man of God; so run from all these evil things. Pursue righteousness and a godly life, along with faith, love, perseverance, and gentleness" (1 Timothy 6:11).

Because Timothy's purpose was to glorify God with his life, he should run from evil and toward God. Our purpose is the same.

The Runner

I never thought I would become a runner. Running was not in my vocabulary. I preferred to walk, ride, or drive to my destination. Instead of playing a sport, I enjoyed sitting on the stands watching the game. Running? For exercise? Never crossed my mind.

And losing weight wasn't an issue for me. I wasn't super skinny, but eating healthy allowed me to stay pretty trim. Running to lose weight? I guess I just never really saw the need for it.

Then something changed.

Recently, in my neighborhood Bible study, we started looking at all the times the Bible used the words *run* or *running*. In Luke 15:11-32, we read about the father running to his prodigal son and discussed what it meant in that culture for a father to run. We read Hebrews 12 and the verses about running the race God has set before us. We also read passages in 1 Timothy and elsewhere that speak about running away from evil.

I wanted to truly understand the meaning of these passages. I was intrigued by all the references to running and wanted to know what it felt like to run—how it challenges, energizes, and develops discipline. Did I really understand what running from evil meant?

Some friends had mentioned that during their runs they would pray and commune with God. At those times of activity and isolation, they could forget their daily stresses and pressures and focus on God.

So I began to run with that purpose. It wasn't easy, but I kept at it and continue because I run to stay close to God, to glorify him.

The Race

Did you notice that Paul used the word *run*? Not *walk* or *saunter* but *run*: move quickly, energetically, and with purpose. What was that purpose? To get away from evil as fast as possible so it wouldn't cause him (and Timothy) to wander off God's path. Paul was not just running

from something, of course; he also was running *toward* something—
a godly life of "faith, love, perseverance, and gentleness."

More than motivating us or keeping us from wandering, having
a purpose also moves us toward our ultimate destination. A purpose
helps us to work through the hard times, to persevere. We learn to
trust in God and to believe that we can change our lives—physically or
spiritually. And as we focus on our ultimate life purpose of glorifying
God, we will be able to fully love and care for the people in our lives.

Paul's letter to Timothy continues: "Fight the good fight for the true
faith. Hold tightly to the eternal life to which God has called you, which
you have confessed so well before many witnesses" (1 Timothy 6:12). As
we run toward a life of godliness, we stay on track by focusing on our
faith and what we believe. If we continue to "run," "pursue," "fight," and
"hold tightly," we will move forward along the path of righteousness and
not wander into sin.

The Result

What is your purpose for running? God calls us to run away from sin
and toward a life filled with faith, love, perseverance, and gentleness.
Are you running in circles, or are you running toward God and his
plan for you? From what sin do you need to run away? Leaving sin isn't
easy, but we must choose to obey with courage and do what is right
so that we may glorify God in all that we do. Get off the sidelines and
have an active faith.

My Story

I had never been the active type, but I started jogging
in college as a way to stay in shape. Since then, God has
transformed my runs into times of worship and conversation
with him. As soon as my shoes hit the asphalt, he invites me
to this place for only me and him. Something about feeling
tired and weak makes it easy to depend on God's strength.

Sometimes I come back from a run in tears because somewhere in between the sweating and aching, God broke my heart for lives with needs bigger than my own. For me, running is good for my body but necessary for my soul.

Tiffany

Think It Through

1. When did you begin running? What got you started?
2. At what times in your running routines do you feel close to God?
3. When has running been a "spiritual experience" for you? What makes it so?
4. What's the difference between "walking" and "running" in your Christian life?

On Running

Does my body type affect my running success?

You can't change your morphology (body build) through exercise and training. Your body composition (the percentage of fat and muscle), however, can change significantly. How does this relate to running success? Well, yes, your body type will affect how effectively you run, but as you run and your body composition changes, your running success will increase.

JOURNAL

_____

_____

_____

_____

_____

_____

RUNNING LOG

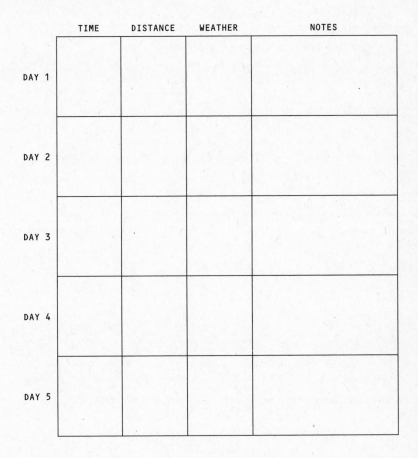

	TIME	DISTANCE	WEATHER	NOTES
DAY 1				
DAY 2				
DAY 3				
DAY 4				
DAY 5				

CREATE A GOAL

You've determined your purpose for running, but you should also have goals. They will provide momentum and push you through the tough times. Your purpose is the big idea—what you hope to achieve long-term. Goals are more immediate and short-term. By setting realistic goals, you will be able to enjoy each run and eventually fulfill your purpose. This doesn't mean, however, that everything will be easy. Yes, goals will help keep you focused, but difficult moments will come. This is true in your spiritual run as well. In preparing young Timothy for his race, Paul explained that he should be prepared for those difficult, sometimes very painful experiences:

> *Endure suffering along with me, as a good soldier of Christ Jesus. Soldiers don't get tied up in the affairs of civilian life, for then they cannot please the officer who enlisted them. And athletes cannot win the prize unless they follow the rules. And hardworking farmers should be the first to enjoy the fruit of their labor. Think about what I am saying. The Lord will help you understand all these things. . . . So I am willing to endure*

anything if it will bring salvation and eternal glory in Christ Jesus to those God has chosen. (2 TIMOTHY 2:3-7, 10)

In this passage, Paul uses the soldier, the farmer, and the athlete as his examples. What do these three people have in common? They have to work hard and "endure suffering" in order to accomplish their goals. The athlete must follow the rules, taking no shortcuts, to reach the finish line. The soldier must leave civilian life and independent living and submit to the officer's commands to have a successful military career. A farmer must till, plant, and weed—hard work—in order to reap a harvest. Paul was in a Roman prison when he wrote that he was "willing to endure anything" to do what God had called him to do. Soon after writing that statement, Paul paid the ultimate price—execution for being a follower of Christ. He suffered, but it was worth it.

Discipline and "suffering" are necessary for more than farmers, soldiers, and athletes. Students need to forgo free-time activities, entertainment options, and sometimes sleep to study for exams or write their essays. Parents have to move their schedules around in order to attend their children's events and sometimes have to scrimp and save for future expenses such as college. Workers sweat and strain, sometimes in terrible conditions, to earn a living.

Christians often must adjust their schedules in order to spend time in the Word, to pray, and to worship. And moved by compassion, they will invest themselves and their resources to help the needy and to spread the gospel. Those choices may seem difficult at the time, but in light of their ultimate purpose (to glorify God), the choices are worth it.

The Runner

I'm exhausted from everything that happened at work today. And the drive home—what a mess. But tonight's the night—the season premiere of four of my favorite TV shows! I have been waiting for this, especially after last season's cliff-hanger, and I'm excited to see what will happen this season. I've been thinking and planning for this night for a while. I even put it on my calendar. Today was crazy, so it will be a nice time to relax.

Yeah, I didn't get my run in, but it's no big deal. I don't think one day will throw me off. I know the race is only two weeks away, but missing today won't hurt my training . . . or will it? I have worked so hard to get to this point, to reach my goal—to run and finish a 10K. I've made it this far because I've stuck to my running schedule, my training plan; otherwise I would be lost and would have given up long ago.

So why am I suddenly distracted and making excuses now? Sure, work was a zoo, and traffic was a beast. And, yes, I would love to sit on the couch and watch my favorite shows. But I'm so close to my goal. And isn't that why we have DVRs?

The Race

Life is filled with potential distractions that can take our focus off our goals. In running, the distractions can include how we're feeling (physical discomforts), other activities (some trivial, like TV shows), the time that running requires, or others' opinions. In our spiritual lives, if we focus on stresses and problems such as job pressures, relationship drama, financial setbacks, and physical needs, the burden of those thoughts will weigh on us and slow us down. We may begin to doubt our capabilities and God's sovereignty. Instead, we must remember that our sufferings build endurance and can bring us closer to God. And we must keep pushing ahead in our spiritual training.

Second Timothy 2:11-12 continues: "If we die with him, we will also live with him. If we endure hardship, we will reign with him." We will reign with him! These trials are only momentary bumps on the road to eternal life with our Lord and Savior, Jesus Christ.

The Result

Instead of focusing on life's complications and struggles, press toward your purpose with the vision of winning and the hope of harvest. God is good. He is here for you. And only through him can you fulfill your ultimate purpose—to glorify God.

What are your goals in your spiritual life? If you decide that you need to have a regular time of Bible study and prayer, a possible goal would be to read and study a book of the Bible by a certain time and to spend thirty minutes a day in this process. If you decide that you need to learn more about Christian doctrine, a possible goal would be to attend one of the adult education classes at your church each time they are offered for a year. Or you may decide to read a couple of the Christian classics. Other goals for spiritual growth, toward fulfilling your purpose of glorifying God, could include getting involved in an outreach, service, tutoring, or other program.

My Story

I hated running. In junior high, I dreaded the mile test. We had to finish in under twelve minutes, and I think I barely made that with my run/walk regimen. Even when I started working out regularly in college, running was not my workout of choice. I'd rather use the elliptical or rowing machine than run.

That's why I'm amazed that within the past couple of years I've completed three triathlons (one as a relay—I was the runner) and numerous road races. It's awesome how God created the human body to push and train itself to reach new goals. I remember struggling to run for a few minutes, but here I am after one year as an "official" runner training for a ten-mile race, a sprint triathlon, and soon a half marathon.

My first race ever was the Chicago Fleet Feet SuperSprint Triathlon (375 meter swim/6.2 mile bike/1.55 mile run). I'd never really trained for anything like this before, and I took it very seriously. On many days, I'd have to get up super early to work out before work, then come home and do another workout. Swimming, biking, and running became my life in addition to an already busy schedule. After I completed the race and had that finisher's medal in my hands, I thought about all the discipline I put into training for the event. How could I be so disciplined to wake up early to swim or run, but when it came to waking up early to read my Bible or spend time with God, I just couldn't do it? The realization convicted me, and I knew I had to change my priorities.

The ultimate race I need to run has spiritual implications. If I want to finish the race God has called me to, then I need to be disciplined in my training for that race by spending time in prayer, reading my Bible, living a life to serve the Lord, etc. In the end, it won't matter how many miles I've run, how many personal records I've set, or how many races I've completed. Only one race matters. So I'll be training, because that's the race I want to finish well.

Christy

Think It Through

1. Without goals, you won't achieve your purpose. What are your current physical/running goals?
2. What are some of your spiritual goals?
3. What goals would help you stay in good spiritual condition?
4. How can you make Christ "real" so that others may see him in you?

On Running

Why should I set goals?

Setting goals has numerous benefits. First, setting goals will help you develop self-confidence as you accomplish them. Second, having goals will motivate you to work harder and be more persistent in your workouts. Third, goal setting will give you insight into your abilities and, hopefully, build your enthusiasm. Finally, working toward achievable goals highlights important aspects of running, helping you improve.

JOURNAL

_____

_____

_____

_____

_____

RUNNING LOG

	TIME	DISTANCE	WEATHER	NOTES
DAY 1				
DAY 2				
DAY 3				
DAY 4				
DAY 5				

CREATE A GOAL

Parents who pray for their children to grow into healthy, caring, and responsible adults should have a series of goals for each of the steps that will get those children to that destination. Students with the ultimate goal or purpose of having a successful career in a chosen field should follow a similar process. Athletes who dream of participating in the Olympics should choose the best path for getting there. We could say the same for any person in any walk of life. *Purpose* refers to the ultimate destination. *Goals* are the hoped-for results for each of the segments on that journey.

In the following passage in 1 Corinthians, Paul used two athletic metaphors—running and boxing—to highlight the necessity of living with purpose. Paul wasn't running just to run, but to get somewhere. He wasn't boxing against the air, but to defeat an opponent. Remembering his purpose and setting his goals helped him discipline himself to train the right way. In this case, Paul wanted to make sure he was living what he preached. Paul's ultimate goal was to glorify God, taking every thought, word, and action captive to the lordship of Christ. So he ran "with purpose in every step."

I run with purpose in every step. I am not just shadowboxing.
I discipline my body like an athlete, training it to do what it
should. Otherwise, I fear that after preaching to others I myself
might be disqualified. (1 CORINTHIANS 9:26-27)

The Runner

Jerome (his friends call him "Romer") is as laid back as they come. He takes life one day, one moment at a time and tends to live totally in the present. That approach has served him well in many cases—he's spontaneous, fun, and creative, and people love his enthusiasm—but it has also held him back in a few areas, especially when he has been expected to meet a deadline at work.

Romer ran track in high school and college—mostly middle distances—so he continued to run after graduation because he liked the feeling before and after his workouts. When Christian friends, guys in his small-group Bible study, asked him to join their team in a marathon and raise money for cancer research in the process, he quickly agreed. As an experienced athlete, Romer knew he would have to train hard to accomplish that goal . . . and he did . . . and *they* did.

At the next Bible study, one of the guys asked what everyone had learned from their marathon experience. A lot was shared, but one lesson hit Jerome as a friend read 1 Corinthians 9:26 and highlighted, "I run with purpose in every step." His friend then explained how training, discipline, and goals relate to living for Christ and said he had determined to consider his spiritual goals so he could run *that* race with purpose too. Jerome decided right then to take what he had learned in training for the marathon and apply it to his faith. He's still good old Romer, up for fun and adventure, but he's now intentional in his spiritual life.

The Race

Anyone who wants to complete a marathon but has no workout plan, including daily goals, will fail. A person can put on the shorts, shirt, socks, and shoes, leave the house, and then just start running, but he or she will probably soon be exhausted and lost. Running with purpose means knowing where you want to go and then developing a plan for getting there.

Paul did not run the race aimlessly, nor was he like someone boxing against air. He ran with purpose, not allowing himself to be lazy or sidetracked. First Corinthians 9:26-27 describes the spiritual maturation process, the period of growth during believers' lives on earth when they are living *in* the world while not being *of* it. The time between a person's trusting Christ as Savior—spiritual birth—and his or her physical death is the only time when spiritual growth can occur. Paul wanted to grow diligently and receive a reward from Christ at his return. Paul did not want to be like the person who builds his or her life with shoddy materials, only to be saved "like someone barely escaping through a wall of flames" (1 Corinthians 3:15).

The Result

What's your spiritual purpose? What do you sense God saying should be your ultimate goal? To be a mature believer, knowing what you believe and living it out? To be a faithful follower of Jesus? After you determine his answer, decide what you need to do to achieve that goal. You may need to spend more time in Bible study and prayer or join a small group or go on a short-term mission trip or help with worship. After determining your goal, you can solidify your plan and get going, running "with purpose in every step."

My Story

After giving birth to my third child, I decided to make a change in my life because I wanted to lose some weight. And we're not talking about a little weight: I wanted to lose sixty pounds. I hadn't exercised at all during my pregnancy and was really out of shape, so how would I ever make this happen?

I belonged to a health club and enjoyed aerobics, but I couldn't put my baby into the club's child-care center until she was six months old. Years earlier, I had gotten somewhat into running. I didn't enjoy it then, but I liked the feeling at the end of my run, and I enjoyed being outside. So I decided running was the only way for me to get moving and lose the weight.

I know my personality and that I need motivation and someone to push me. That's one thing I've enjoyed about aerobics classes—having an instructor who will encourage me and hold me accountable. If I were really going to run regularly, I would need a goal. A big one. A half-marathon race was being held nearby in a few months . . . could I do it?

I called my sister, a runner, to find out if it was even possible to train in three months to run 13.1 miles. She created a training plan, and three months later the two of us crossed the finish line together.

I met my goal of the half marathon, and you know what else? I got in shape and lost weight—my purpose for running.

Kara

Think It Through

1. What's the farthest you've run? What's the longest race you've entered?
2. What did you have to do to reach your running goal for that race?
3. What's your biggest spiritual challenge right now?
4. What steps do you need to take to meet that challenge?

On Running

How do I set goals?

First of all, consider your ultimate purpose, because reaching your goals should help you achieve that purpose. Next, assess your abilities and needs.

Be realistic, but make sure that you don't underestimate yourself. Where do you need the most help with running? Is it motivation? Do you want to run faster? Do you want your legs to be less tired? Be sure to set goals in a variety of areas. Don't just focus on distance, but look at intensity and mind frame. Then identify the factors that will affect your goals: time, commitment, and abilities. Finally, develop a realistic plan that will help you to reach your goals.

JOURNAL

_____

_____

_____

_____

_____

_____

_____

_____

_____

_____

_____

_____

_____

_____

_____

_____

_____

_____

_____

_____

RUNNING LOG

	TIME	DISTANCE	WEATHER	NOTES
DAY 1				
DAY 2				
DAY 3				
DAY 4				
DAY 5				

DEVELOP A PLAN

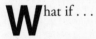hat if . . .

- a construction worker, right off the site, started as offensive tackle for the New Orleans Saints?
- a recent college graduate was named CEO of General Electric?
- a driver's education student decided to drive an eighteen-wheeler from Dallas to Minneapolis?
- an athletic trainer wanted to perform brain surgery?

Ridiculous, of course . . . with no good endings. In each case, the individual would need training and practice to achieve the desired level of competence. And that doesn't just happen—moving from point A (idea/dream) to point Z (accomplishment) takes a plan, a thoughtful and practical step-by-step process. Training and practice are certainly necessary with running success. Anyone can buy a nice outfit, register, get a number, show up at the starting line, cheer when the gun goes off, and maybe even run a mile or two. But only those who have trained by putting in the months and miles will finish the marathon.

That's the point of Hebrews 5:14, too, which says, "Solid food is for those who are mature, who through training have the skill to recognize the difference between right and wrong." Babies don't suddenly chomp on steak. They begin with milk; then, as they grow and develop, they eventually become mature enough physically to handle solid food. Baby believers (new Christians) also need to begin with baby steps. As they grow and train, eventually they mature to where they can "recognize the difference between right and wrong." To go from A to Z in the spiritual life also takes a plan, a training schedule.

The Runner

She wanted to run. She really did, especially after seeing how much her friends seemed to enjoy the experience, not to mention their weight loss. In her midthirties, she knew she ought to have a regular exercise program for her health and to keep her weight down. So that Wednesday in September she decided to go for it, and she signed up for the Turkey Trot, a 5K race just before Thanksgiving. The next day she bought shoes, shorts, and socks at the running store. And after work on Friday she went for a run around the block a couple of times. *That wasn't so bad*, she thought, and a few days later she tried it again. She figured she would run every other day, usually in the afternoons. But with the daylight hours decreasing and the temps going down, she missed a day here and there, especially when she had to work late. On the big day, she drove to the park and walked to the starting line, eagerly anticipating her first race! Caught up in the excitement, she began fast and ran well for the first half mile or so. But after a mile she was gassed. So she quit . . . frustrated and disappointed with herself.

The Race

Like the woman in the story, many people can't reach their goal, so they quit. Others give up running even sooner than she did. They go out and run and are soon exhausted. Maybe they even try that approach a few times, but then they decide they can't do it and hang up their shoes. In both cases, the runners don't succeed because they run without a plan. Unlike other aerobic activities, building running endurance can be a slow process. Being able to jump out of bed, throw on sweats, lace up the shoes, and go for a quick five-mile run (never having worked out) would be nice, but that's not reality. On the other hand, with a training plan anyone without serious physical limitations can become a runner. The plan takes you from point A to point Z, helping you reach your goal and your purpose for running in the first place.

The spiritual parallel is obvious. A young follower of Christ may dream about being able to preach or teach the Bible the way pastors do. That's a worthy goal, but to reach it will take many hours (perhaps years) of study and training. Or a new believer may want to understand the deeper issues of the faith—again a worthy goal, but reaching it will take time and a plan. Even those who have been Christians for many years need to continue to grow in the faith. In fact, the apostle Peter says, "Those who fail to develop in this way are shortsighted or blind, forgetting that they have been cleansed from their old sins" (2 Peter 1:9).

To reach those goals takes a plan.

The Result

A spiritual-growth plan needs to be a daily "workout" of spending time reading the Bible and praying. The plan also should include regular worship and teaching, at church and other venues. And we must not forget community—building strong relationships with other believers. In the process, we should look for ways to serve, to use our gifts and meet needs inside and outside the church. God will provide many opportunities for growth: teaching, preaching, worshiping, serving, giving, and faith-stretching. And we should take advantage of those. But we need to be intentional, praying about, thinking through, and living out a plan to reach those spiritual goals.

My Story

"The prudent understand where they are going" (Proverbs 14:8).

I've always seen the value in planning ahead, even when it comes to my running routine. Most nights before an early-morning run, I lay out my running apparel, GPS watch, iPod, sunglasses, water bottle, and house key. I find it helpful to pray about the next day's run and ask God for endurance and strength and to help me enjoy my running time. When preparing for a race, I plan ahead by registering early and mapping a chart for improving and beating my previous chip time.

Not only does planning help me to be more efficient with my busy schedule, it also keeps me committed to following through with my training. If I don't plan ahead, I'm more likely to sleep in and blow off my runs, and therefore I fail to honor my commitment to keep up with my training schedule.

That's sort of the way it is with serving and honoring the Lord. It's easy to get lazy when you don't have a good plan in place. God is totally committed to us for a lifetime, and nothing can break that commitment. When we give our time to God through serving others, praying, and reading the Bible, we show our commitment to him. And when we include God in our plans, we know that his ultimate purpose will prevail.

Becky B.

Think It Through

1. How did you develop your running plan?
2. What steps do you need to take on the road to spiritual maturity, or even to put yourself back on God's path?
3. Considering your spiritual goals, what are the first three steps you need to take to get from here to there?

4. What resources do you need (for example, Bible, study tools, local church, class, etc.)? Where can you find those?

On Running

What should I eat before running?

If you eat before you run, you should do it three to five hours beforehand to allow your food to digest and to keep you from a quick sugar response that can lead to an energy crash. The amount you eat doesn't really matter. Eating before a run or competition replenishes your glycogen stores—your easily accessible energy.

JOURNAL

_____

_____

_____

_____

_____

_____

_____

_____

_____

_____

_____

RUNNING LOG

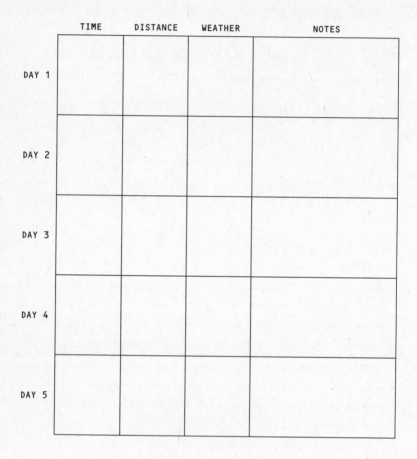

	TIME	DISTANCE	WEATHER	NOTES
DAY 1				
DAY 2				
DAY 3				
DAY 4				
DAY 5				

DEVELOP A PLAN

You're probably familiar with Jesus' parables recorded in Matthew 13, especially the first one about the sower, seeds, and soils. Jesus explained the parable's meaning to the disciples, and he ended with this statement: "The seed that fell on good soil represents those who truly hear and understand God's word and produce a harvest of thirty, sixty, or even a hundred times as much as had been planted!" (Matthew 13:23). Upon hearing this, we can imagine the disciples thinking, *Wow—a hundredfold return!* They had signed on to follow Jesus because they believed in him and his message, and they understood that their purpose on earth was to spread the Good News about the Kingdom of God. Thus, they might have taken Jesus' words about the result of sowing seeds on good soil to mean guaranteed success. So Jesus followed with another parable—this one about wheat and weeds:

> *The Kingdom of Heaven is like a farmer who planted good seed in his field. But that night as the workers slept, his enemy came and planted weeds among the wheat, then slipped away. When the crop began to grow and produce grain, the weeds also grew.*

The farmer's workers went to him and said, "Sir, the field where you planted that good seed is full of weeds! Where did they come from?"

"An enemy has done this!" the farmer exclaimed.

"Should we pull out the weeds?" they asked.

"No," he replied, "you'll uproot the wheat if you do. Let both grow together until the harvest. Then I will tell the harvesters to sort out the weeds, tie them into bundles, and burn them, and to put the wheat in the barn." (MATTHEW 13:24-30)

Jesus' clear message was that as the disciples were out sowing gospel seeds, Satan would be sowing weeds. In other words, they shouldn't expect the process to be easy. As they developed their ministry plan, they needed to have the right—realistic—expectations.

In another passage, Jesus put it this way:

Don't begin until you count the cost. For who would begin construction of a building without first calculating the cost to see if there is enough money to finish it? Otherwise, you might complete only the foundation before running out of money, and then everyone would laugh at you. They would say, "There's the person who started that building and couldn't afford to finish it!" (LUKE 14:28-30)

Your plans for spiritual growth and for running need to be realistic, taking into account all sorts of possibilities.

The Runner

Ethan had it all figured out. The marathon was scheduled for mid-November, so he would begin his training regimen three months before, making sure to follow the schedule laid out in the running magazine. He did really well at first—the shorter runs weren't very tough and didn't take much time . . . and the weather was okay for August, not too hot or humid. But an unseasonably hot week in September knocked him off stride a bit, and the wind and rain in October made running really tough. So before long he was a week behind in his training schedule . . . and then two. Pressures at work didn't help either; the longer days at the office and a couple of sales trips meant less time for those long runs. As for the marathon, Ethan finished, struggling desperately through the last 10K, but his time was way off his goal—all because he hadn't been able to put in the miles.

The problem? Ethan's plan was riddled with idealistic assumptions.

The Race

Some people get the idea that if they trust in Christ, all their problems will disappear; they'll be prosperous and popular, healthy and heroic. That assumption would be like expecting to breeze through a marathon, and the letdown would be similar when challenges come. You may be ready physically for the run, but you might awaken feeling woozy, race day might be hot and humid, and the course might be pocked with potholes and almost invisible bumps (surprise!). In other words, you may discover that your plan was far from reality. A much better approach is to be prepared for unexpected problems and issues, having a good supply of nutrients, water, petroleum gel, and bandages ready and nearby if you need them. Just running 26.2 miles can be a painful ordeal without having to deal with blisters, chafing, and dehydration. Idealism and impatience will create many more problems than they solve.

The Result

God has given us many positive promises in his Word concerning success, joy, and hope. But he also clearly states that the way will be rough. We need to be prepared for those difficult times, with spiritual salves and bandages and a support team. Jesus told his disciples, "I have told you all this so that you may have peace in me. Here on earth you will have many trials and sorrows. But take heart, because I have overcome the world" (John 16:33). We need to plan and plan well. And here's the great news: The Christian race won't be easy, but we're not running alone—our Lord is running with us.

My Story

At the end of my sophomore year of high school, rumors were flying that my school was establishing a girls' soccer team the following year. When the rumors became reality, I was elated. When it was subsequently announced that tryouts would involve sprints, fartleks (a form of interval training developed in Sweden), and a timed one-mile run, I was slightly discouraged, but I remained grounded in my purpose. I was determined to make the summer before my junior year my inauguration into the world of running.

In my imaginings of what this particular summer of running would involve, I envisioned my nonrunner self tying my shoelaces for that first run, and then I pictured my end-of-summer self—toned, fast, ready for soccer. My failure was in ignoring the actual running part: the physical exertion, the aching muscles, the lack of oxygen reaching my brain. It took me about thirty seconds of my first run to realize that this was going to be a long summer.

Desperate times called for desperately pathetic measures. I made a plan: run two minutes, walk two minutes. Once I had mastered that, I decided to run for the duration of one song on my iPod. The song lasted about four minutes, and as it was finishing, I felt like I was on top of the world. Then the song actually finished, and I almost threw up. When summer ended, the cross-country team was nice enough to let me train with them without competing in actual races.

The pain and the time and the feeling of being ridiculously slow were worth it. I made the soccer team—and was named junior captain. I was still slow and steady, but maybe my coach knew the girls at the rear of the pack during our practices needed more encouragement from their leader than the girls sprinting at the front. And in a way, isn't that just like God's upside-down Kingdom? He seems to have a habit of placing "the least" of his Kingdom in positions of unexpected honor. The surprising irony of God is so meaningful to the slow and steady among us.

Sarah

Think It Through

1. How have you factored into your running plan possible difficulties (weather, health, responsibilities, etc.)?
2. When did you realize that being a Christian doesn't keep you from pain and problems?
3. How have you factored into your spiritual plan possible difficulties (economic stress, physical challenges, relationship drama, etc.)?
4. What support team do you have in place to come alongside you during those tough times and spiritual struggles?

On Running

What are the different types of goals?

With a *subjective* goal, the intent is on having fun and doing your best. *Objective* goals develop a standard of proficiency for a task within an allotted time. *Outcome*-oriented goals focus on achieving victory in a competitive situation. *Performance* goals focus on achieving standards based on your own previous performances rather than others' standards. Finally, *process* goals focus on the action of the activity itself in order to properly execute a skill.

JOURNAL

_____

_____

_____

_____

_____

RUNNING LOG

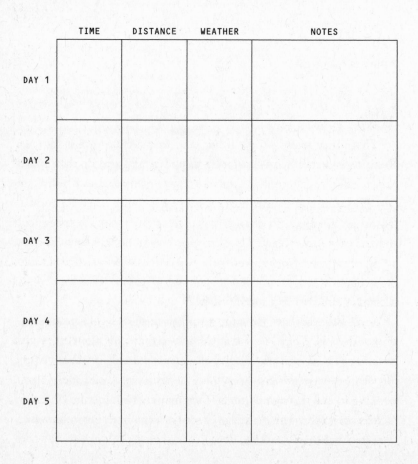

	TIME	DISTANCE	WEATHER	NOTES
DAY 1				
DAY 2				
DAY 3				
DAY 4				
DAY 5				

GET ADVICE

What could be difficult or complicated about running? You just lace up the shoes and take off!

That's how many people think, and to a certain extent it's true. Running is certainly much simpler to understand and do than sports such as tennis, golf, football, speed skating, gymnastics, or mountain climbing. But that doesn't mean it's easy, especially when longer distances are involved. So getting advice from experts and experienced runners only makes sense. They can give insight and guidance in every aspect of running, from choosing the right shoes to knowledge of training programs and plans. And imagine what we can learn from those who have already run a specific route.

Some believers have the same simplistic approach to their relationship with God. They know that salvation is by faith alone; they just have to trust in Christ to forgive their sins and to give them eternal life. And they know that everything depends on God's Holy Spirit working in and through them. So they may try running the Christian race on their own, with no outside input or help. In doing so, however, they may be unprepared for what lies in their path, or they may take a wrong turn. The Bible offers several encouragements to listen and learn from others, as well as warnings about false teachers who will try to lead us astray.

Friends, experts, and wise counselors can help in running and in life. Proverbs highlights that truth: "Plans go wrong for lack of advice; many advisers bring success" (Proverbs 15:22).

The Runner

Megan never saw herself as an athlete. She had participated in the usual childhood sports—soccer, swimming, gymnastics—but hadn't even tried out for school teams in junior and senior high school. So when she decided to run, she knew she needed good advice. The first person she asked was Kelli, a friend from church and an experienced runner. Kelli told Megan about the importance of finding the right shoes and suggested a store where the salespeople knew what they were talking about. Kelli also gave tips on stretching, pacing, fluid intake, and how to deal with blisters, chafing, and other aches and pains. Megan subscribed to a running magazine and looked for information on the Internet.

Running wasn't easy for Megan, but she took the advice of Kelli and others, designed a plan, and achieved her running goals.

The Race

Getting wise counsel (and heeding it) makes sense in every area of life, not just running. Only foolish or prideful people think they know enough to be successful in anything they try with no help from anyone. So why do we often try to live the Christian life on our own? Anyone planning a trip to another country certainly would read about the country and the insights from travel pros, and they'd talk with friends who had traveled there previously. The traveler would want to know about packing, overcoming jet lag, currency, safety, customs, and not-to-miss sites and experiences. The faith parallels are obvious: Believers need counsel for this trip, in this race.

We can find these counselors at church—mature believers who know the journey. They can answer what-to-do-when questions and can guide us toward success and away from failure. They can also confront us when necessary and challenge us to make godly choices. Paul wrote to the Ephesian believers about the importance of working together and learning from each other: "Now these are the gifts Christ gave to the church: the apostles, the prophets, the evangelists, and the pastors and teachers. Their responsibility is to equip God's people to do his work and build up the church, the body of Christ" (Ephesians 4:11-12).

The Result

The Christian life is a marathon, not a sprint, so you'll need wise counsel to help you plan and prepare for the race. Along the way you will encounter twists and turns in the course and unexpected obstacles and other challenges, so you'll need wise advice on how to respond. And you'll even meet those who would try to mislead you and get you off course, so you'll need help in determining the right way to go. Remember, "many advisers" (the right advisers) "bring success."

My Story

I had been running for several years, beginning with high school cross-country. So I was pretty confident in my knowledge of the sport. In college, I had run to stay in shape and had competed in several 5K and 10K races. So I thought I'd try the big one—a marathon. I followed a good workout schedule and knew I was ready as the race approached.

My dad, also an avid runner who had run a few marathons, tried to give me some advice. He said to taper the last week before the race, get a good night's sleep, eat something, and be sure to take fluids early on because I would need them later. But I did just the opposite: I didn't get much rest, I didn't eat anything that morning because I thought it would slow me down, I ran by all the early aid stations because I didn't want to feel bloated and thought I would feel the drink sloshing around.

What a mistake! Just before the twenty-mile marker, I hit the wall . . . hard. And I struggled to even finish, limping, walking, shuffling to the end. My father knew me, and he knew running—if only I had listened to his advice. In my next marathon, I followed his suggestions and finished one hour faster!

Elizabeth

Think It Through

1. What advice resources are you aware of for running (people, coaches, magazines, websites, etc.)? How will you use them to help you plan, prepare for, and reach your running goals?
2. Who are your spiritual counselors/advisers? How are they involved in helping you meet your spiritual goals?
3. Where will you go for advice on dealing with temptation and sin? How about relationship issues?
4. Where will you go for counsel and guidance in knowing whether a teacher or teaching is true or false?

On Running

Should I eat anything while running?

If your run is less than an hour, you will have no need to eat anything while running—it's not very beneficial. For a longer event, you will want a way to replace carbohydrates every fifteen minutes. Some options might be a sports drink at the beginning. The longer the race, the more you might want to increase the amount of carbohydrates. Orange slices are good—they are light on the stomach and provide some good energy. For long races like marathons, different types of compacted gel carbohydrates provide a big punch of energy. Be sure, however, to drink plenty of water when consuming the gel.

JOURNAL

_____

_____

_____

_____

_____

RUNNING LOG

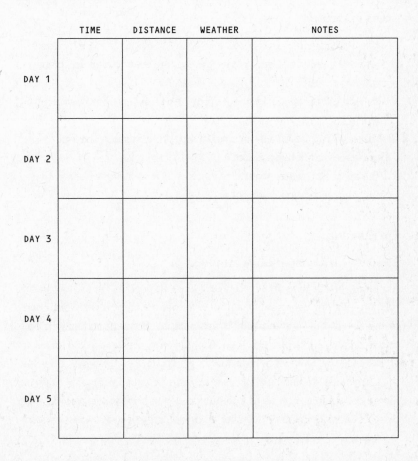

	TIME	DISTANCE	WEATHER	NOTES
DAY 1				
DAY 2				
DAY 3				
DAY 4				
DAY 5				

GET ADVICE

Counsel and input from friends and fellow runners is valuable, but imagine getting long-distance running advice from Haile Gebrselassie from Ethiopia (men's marathon world record holder—2:03:59, set in 2008) or Paula Radcliffe from Great Britain (women's marathon world record holder—2:15:25, set in 2003). Who we listen to makes a big difference.

The same is true in the Christian life. But here's a huge difference: Obtaining the services of a world-class runner or coach would be virtually impossible, but believers can learn from the ultimate spiritual Coach. In fact, he—our Creator and Redeemer, almighty God—invites us to talk with him and to read his playbook, the Bible. Yet many believers take for granted his presence or ignore his guidance. Not a good move.

The psalm writer Asaph declares, "You guide me with your counsel, leading me to a glorious destiny" (Psalm 73:24). He knew where following God's advice would lead . . . and he followed.

The Runner

Troy swam competitively at the collegiate level and would swim laps at the Y pool a few times a week. He also had been riding his bike for a few years, so he was in good physical condition. But Troy had decided to compete in the local triathlon and needed to add running to his workout routine. (Eventually, he would like to finish an Ironman triathlon.) He wanted to do it right, so he researched online and talked with every runner he knew.

After a couple of weeks, Troy was pretty sure he could lay out a plan for successfully competing, except for one problem: Some of the advice from his runner friends seemed contradictory. One person told him to stretch for a long time before and after running; another one said that stretching wasn't necessary, and he shouldn't waste the time. And the advice varied on everything from the right shoes to buy to proper race pacing. Then, while reading the paper, he learned that a world-class marathon runner would be holding a clinic in another town. So he drove the hour, listened to the runner, and was able to spend some time with the runner one-on-one and ask all his questions. Good move!

The Race

We don't have to drive an hour to talk with our Expert on faith and life—we can turn to him anytime in prayer. And we can easily access his book. So why don't we do that more often? We may be so busy that one-on-one time with him gets crowded out of the schedule. We may think we've done all that before and take his guidance for granted. Or we may be unsure how to read and understand his Word. Fortunately, we have hundreds of resources available to us: modern language Bible translations (for example, the New Living Translation), study Bibles (for example, the *Life Application Study Bible*), commentaries and other Bible study tools, devotionals (such as this one), and many others in various formats. And we can hear Bible teachers through TV, the radio, CDs, the Internet, and podcasts. In addition, our other spiritual advisers can direct us to Bible passages and help explain their meaning and application.

The Result

God wants us to run his race right, to successfully complete the course, and he's given everything we need in his Word. We just need to read, study, and apply it. The apostle Paul writes:

All Scripture is inspired by God and is useful to teach us what is true and to make us realize what is wrong in our lives. It corrects us when we are wrong and teaches us to do what is right. God uses it to prepare and equip his people to do every good work.
(2 TIMOTHY 3:16-17)

Get advice from the One who knows.

My Story

In the mid 1980s, I ran a 5K road race in LaGrange, Illinois. Four of us were bunched in a group behind the lead runner. The rest of the field was far behind us. All I had to do was hold on and I would have no worse than fifth place. That is, if the fellow standing on the corner giving directions had pointed correctly. As Bugs Bunny said, "Nyahhh, I should've taken that left turn at Albuquerque." We soon realized the problem, but none of us knew the area. A 3.1-mile race turned into a 5.5-mile run. We all finished near last place. Lesson learned? Check the map and be ready to run as long as needed.

Anthony

Think It Through

1. How many Bibles do you own? Which one do you read most often?
2. What keeps you from having a regular time of Bible study and prayer?
3. What study tools do you need to help you understand and apply Scripture?
4. What running buddy or other friend can you enlist to hold you accountable for this spiritual discipline?

On Running

How does my body stay cool in the heat?

Your body can stay cool in the heat in four ways: radiation, conduction, convection, and evaporation. Radiation is the vibration of heat molecules off skin and into the atmosphere. This accounts for 60 percent of heat loss. Conduction is direct contact with something cooler—your body gives off heat to that object. Convection is the movement of one medium across the skin surface (wind blowing, etc.). Finally, evaporation (found only in humans) occurs when the body sweats, and the evaporation of the sweat cools off the skin.

JOURNAL

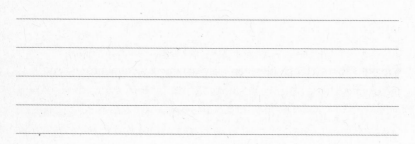

RUNNING LOG

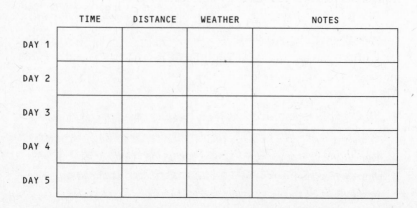

	TIME	DISTANCE	WEATHER	NOTES
DAY 1				
DAY 2				
DAY 3				
DAY 4				
DAY 5				

GEAR UP

In any sport, having the right equipment is crucial; sometimes it can make the difference between success and failure, winning and losing. Again, this is obvious in sports such as ice hockey, football, skiing, cycling, and kayaking, in which competitors wear a variety of pads or depend on something they must ride, pedal, or paddle. In a sport such as running, we might assume that the "equipment," what little there is, has little if any impact on performance. What a mistake! Everything from shoes to shirts can make a huge difference.

The Bible often uses the metaphor of putting on clothes to picture various aspects of the Christian life. In both cases—running and living for Christ—having the right equipment is crucial. Consider Paul's message to the Roman believers:

> *The night is almost gone; the day of salvation will soon be here. So remove your dark deeds like dirty clothes, and put on the shining armor of right living. Because we belong to the day, we must live decent lives for all to see. Don't participate in the darkness of wild parties and drunkenness, or in sexual*

promiscuity and immoral living, or in quarreling and jealousy.
Instead, clothe yourself with the presence of the Lord Jesus Christ.
And don't let yourself think about ways to indulge your evil
desires. (ROMANS 13:12-14)

The Runner

He was ready for the marathon (his first), having put in more than
three months of miles. Carefully following the workout schedule laid
out in the running magazine, he had eventually completed two twenty-
mile runs. The only problem, as he could see it, was that his shoes were
getting worn and ratty—would they even hold up? So he went to the
running store and bought a good pair with a nice, cushiony feel. While
there, he also bought a new running outfit. Then he wore the shoes the
last week before the race, to break them in, as he eased off on distance
(and loaded up on carbohydrates).

Early on the morning of the marathon, he put on the new running
shirt, shorts, socks, and shoes, and headed for the start. The gun went
off, and our runner disciplined himself to keep his pace, confident in
his new shoes. At about six miles, however, he began to feel it—chafing
on the collar and arms of his new shirt and blisters forming on his feet.
He stopped to apply Vaseline, but that only gave relief for a couple of
miles. At about the ten-mile mark, every stride was painful . . . and he
had sixteen more to go! At twelve miles he gave up, barely able to walk,
let alone run . . . defeated by his shoes.

The Race

Experienced runners know that wearing the right equipment for a
marathon, especially shoes, is crucial. Imagine someone showing up to
the starting line wearing jeans and sandals and expecting to compete.
The person may be able to run a few yards, perhaps even make a mile,
but he or she would be in terrible shape. The continual pounding and
moving of the legs and arms over long distances will magnify any rub

or irritation. For example, a tag on the back of a shirt or shorts can rub away the skin, and shoes that are a bit tight or loose in certain places can cause serious blisters or other issues. They should be chosen carefully—with consideration given to the runner's weight, stride, and step—and thoroughly broken in before the race. The best-looking shoes may turn out to be the worst choice.

For the Christian race, Paul urges believers to wear the "shining armor of right living" and to be clothed with the presence of the Lord Jesus Christ. But before lacing up *those* shoes and shorts, we need to get rid of the old ones, which Paul calls our "dark deeds." Then he gets specific, warning against the "darkness of wild parties and drunkenness, . . . sexual promiscuity and immoral living, . . . quarreling and jealousy." Those old clothes will hinder us in this race. We need to gear up!

The Result

Some try to keep up Christian appearances while harboring secret "dark deeds." But anyone who wants to run the real race must remove those clothes, that old life, and put on the equipment provided by our heavenly Coach. These are lifestyle choices. God has told you what to do, how to live. The choice is yours.

My Story

I love walking into the running store on a mission, whether that means buying new running shoes, cold weather running tights, an armband to hold my iPhone, or even a few new packs of GU Energy Gel for my long runs—it is a magical feeling! Why? I think because when I have the right gear, my goal seems more attainable.

I feel "fit" in my favorite running outfit and actually run faster. Without properly fitting running shoes, one can never put in the long miles. A shoe that works for me won't necessarily work for someone else because we are all so different in the size and shape of our feet, the way we run, our posture, our heel strike, etc. One size does not fit all when it comes to running!

Having the right gear for those long runs correlates directly to having the right gear for my faith journey and the race that God wants me to run. When I began running, I had very little faith, no strong Christian values, and no idea that God had a plan for me. I attribute this dark point in my life to not having the proper "gear." Oh, I had the right running shoes, cute clothes, and water bottles, but I was lacking the proper gear for my Christian walk of life and the real race I should have been training for. It was only after I "geared up" with the essentials—which included a loving, Christian husband; a church and small group to help keep me accountable; reading God's Word through the Bible and devotionals; daily prayer; Christian music; and Christian community—that I fully understood that God had a plan for me and that this is his race.

With the right gear we can properly train, race, and attain our goals. I also need to have the right gear in my day-to-day life. The company I keep, the books I read, and the music I listen to all help shape my day and my journey with God. This "armor" of God helps me to stay focused on what he wants for me and protects me from outside forces that want to pull me away from him. Just like my cold-weather running gear protects me from the elements, my Christian gear protects me from the devil himself.

Ellen

Think It Through

1. What spiritual "running clothes" do you need to get rid of?
2. Why is this so difficult to do?
3. What does your new, spiritual running equipment look like, your "shining armor of right living"?
4. How can you be assured of the "presence of the Lord Jesus Christ"?

On Running

What should I wear when running in the heat?

Because your body needs to get rid of heat quickly, you shouldn't wear too many clothes. In order to release heat by convection, the body needs to be open to the air. Running attire made of cotton is not a good choice because cotton absorbs and holds sweat. Instead, look for shirts and shorts made of fabric that wicks away sweat, allowing the body to cool itself through evaporation. Not only will you not get as hot, but your clothing won't be as heavy!

JOURNAL

RUNNING LOG

	TIME	DISTANCE	WEATHER	NOTES
DAY 1				
DAY 2				
DAY 3				
DAY 4				
DAY 5				

GEAR UP

Having the correct basic equipment for a sport is important, but equally important is having that equipment available for different aspects of a contest or for conditions that might arise. In football, players might have to change their spikes for a better grip in mud or even change into different shoes altogether when playing on an icy surface. Baseball players need sunglasses that they can quickly flip down when trying to track a pop-up or fly ball in the bright sky. And NASCAR owners and drivers understand that their tires will vary depending on track conditions.

So how do runners cope with ice, wind, rain, sun, and other race circumstances? They are geared up with the right equipment.

As Christ-followers, we also need to be prepared for a wide variety of life possibilities and situations. Although Paul wasn't talking to runners, he challenged believers in Ephesus to don the right equipment—armor for their spiritual battle. They needed to be dressed from head to toe in order to meet the onslaughts of the enemy, Satan himself:

A final word: Be strong in the Lord and in his mighty power.
Put on all of God's armor so that you will be able to stand firm

against all strategies of the devil. For we are not fighting against flesh-and-blood enemies, but against evil rulers and authorities of the unseen world, against mighty powers in this dark world, and against evil spirits in the heavenly places.

Therefore, put on every piece of God's armor so you will be able to resist the enemy in the time of evil. Then after the battle you will still be standing firm. Stand your ground, putting on the belt of truth and the body armor of God's righteousness. For shoes, put on the peace that comes from the Good News so that you will be fully prepared. In addition to all of these, hold up the shield of faith to stop the fiery arrows of the devil. Put on salvation as your helmet, and take the sword of the Spirit, which is the word of God. (EPHESIANS 6:10-17).

The Runner

For René's marathon, the race-day weather forecast was foreboding—cold (thirty-five degrees Fahrenheit), misty rain, and wind. Eventually, however, the rain would stop, the sun would break through, and the temperature would climb—at least that's what the meteorologist said. So René laid out her running clothes, everything she would need.

Her objective was to be as light as possible while also retaining body heat; thus, layering was in order. Next to her body would be her basic running outfit—lightweight, smooth, and loose. Over that, she would put on a short-sleeve T-shirt, and over that a long-sleeve shirt. Then she grabbed a garbage bag that she would tear holes in and wear over everything. It was light, cheap, and easily discarded. On her hands, she would wear old sweat socks. These would allow her to ball up her fingers to keep them warm, and she wouldn't mind losing the socks at the right time. René also wanted to keep her head covered, so she took her running hat with the built-in sweat band, and she covered it with plastic that she could rip off if she wanted. As far as her legs were concerned, René knew that they would warm up quickly, so she wouldn't need to cover them for the race. She would wear her sweat pants until just before the start, when she would take them off and hand them to a friend.

The Race

Serious runners understand that running conditions will not always be ideal, especially if they travel and run in varying climates. Fortunately, sporting-goods manufacturers have developed equipment to help runners adapt to and run in almost any weather and on virtually all terrain. The key is to think ahead and be prepared for workouts and races.

God has given Christians everything needed for running and winning the race of faith. All the gear is available, ready for us to use. We just have to put it on so we'll be prepared. Using the metaphor of fighting a battle, Paul describes the armor-equipment we'll need and what each piece represents: belt (truth), body armor (righteousness), shoes (peace from the Good News), shield (faith), helmet (salvation), and sword (Word of God). Paul makes two main points: First, we're in a battle, not at a picnic; second, we need to be ready, to be geared up.

In effect, Paul is saying we'll be prepared if we are assured of our relationship with God, knowing that we have settled the salvation issue (helmet), that God is truth, and that we have the truth (belt). Standing firm on the truth of the gospel (shoes), we move with confidence and in faith (shield), living the way God wants (body armor) and striking out with Scripture (sword) against the forces of evil.

The Result

Serious followers of Christ know they must be grounded in God's Word. Satan likes to attack our assurance, sowing doubts. He has used this trick since the beginning, when he asked Eve, "Did God really say you must not eat the fruit from any of the trees in the garden?"

(Genesis 3:1). He whispers questions about our salvation, the inspiration of Scripture, the uniqueness of Christ, and even the existence of God. When we fail to wear the helmet and belt, we become vulnerable to other temptations.

Satan's distractions and temptations aren't the only potential race conditions, of course. We will also face physical, relational, financial, and emotional challenges.

Every day, put on your equipment and run your race with confidence, prepared for anything Satan or anyone else can throw at you.

My Story

I have learned so much about running as I have grown older. In high school I ran cross-country and track. In those competitions the ultimate goal was to run faster and win, so that was how I was conditioned. I was a decent competitor but never actually liked running, only the social part of it. In college I stopped running because it wasn't fun. Quite honestly, it was torture at its finest. I didn't actually pick it up again until I was in my thirties.

One day, as I was leaving the YMCA after a fitness class, I noticed a group of eight to ten women dressed for the cold and getting ready to brave the Chicago wind. It was the Y Running Club, and I immediately knew I had to become a part of it. I wasn't sure why, but I was completely interested. I began running with the group and over the course of the year learned that running is so much more than just *running*. I loved the women and the social aspect of running, but I discovered so many technicalities.

For example, I discovered that "pacing" doesn't always mean taking off at breakneck speed. I also learned the importance of stretching and strength training so I could not only increase my speed but also stay healthy and run happily.

As for attire, I learned that looking cute in the
winter isn't important, but staying warm is; thus,
clothing choice is crucial to a happy run. I had never
lived above the Mason-Dixon Line, so winter running
attire for me meant a long-sleeve cotton T-shirt and
sweats. My first run in a Chicago winter was a wake-up
call. I was ill prepared and suffered the consequences.
I needed a day to thaw out and was fortunate not to
have caught pneumonia.

I have found that my spiritual life parallels my
running life. I cannot survive all that life throws
at me without the proper attire. I've learned that in
Chicago I need layers while running in the cold. I start
with a skintight base layer and put a warmer layer over
it. Up top, I wear a couple of layers under a specialty
zip-up fleece that combats the wind. I have warmer socks
for winter and hats and gloves to finish off the outfit.
It is impossible to run *happily*—without the proper gear.

Similarly, it is hard to live *happily* without God's
gear, his "armor." Over the last few years, our family
has dealt with the impossible. Our six-year-old son,
Max, was diagnosed with a rare brain tumor in October
2008 and died July 4, 2009. During our journey, we
learned not only to trust in God's plan for our lives
but to put on his armor every day to combat whatever
Satan threw our way.

In Ephesians 6:10-18, Paul tells Christians to put on
the belt of truth, the body armor of righteousness, feet
fitted with readiness, the shield of faith, the helmet
of salvation, and the sword of the Spirit, praying in
the Spirit constantly. We have learned that nothing is
impossible with God. On some days I can't put on the
armor—that's when I ask God to put it on for me. God's
love and peace have gotten me through so much in running
. . . and in life.

Leanne

Think It Through

1. What piece of spiritual running gear do you need the most?
2. When have you been most vulnerable to those whispers of doubt about your faith?
3. What other conditions do you think you will face in your spiritual race?
4. What should you do to be better prepared for them?

On Running

How should I prepare for running in the heat?

When running in heat and humidity, you can take steps to keep from over-heating. First, be sure to hyper-hydrate; in other words, drink plenty of water before beginning your run and drink during the run. Second, begin at a slower pace (not your race pace) so your body can adjust to the heat. Also, maintain a slightly slower pace throughout your workout. If you wear a heart-rate monitor, you will be able to keep track of your workout and see when you need to slow down. Finally, the best help for running in hotter-than-normal conditions is acclimatization. Just six to ten days in hot and humid weather will help your body to adjust and become used to the heat.

JOURNAL

_____

_____

_____

_____

_____

_____

_____

RUNNING LOG

	TIME	DISTANCE	WEATHER	NOTES
DAY 1				
DAY 2				
DAY 3				
DAY 4				
DAY 5				

ESTABLISH A ROUTINE

What's your daily routine? If you have a job, during the week you may follow a general schedule such as this: wake up, get ready, eat, drive to work, work, drive home, eat dinner, relax, go to bed. Sometimes you probably wish you could live moment to moment, simply doing what you feel like at any given time, ignoring deadlines, responsibilities, and appointments. That kind of spontaneous living may be fun, but you know it wouldn't work—you certainly wouldn't keep your job very long. While routines can be, well, routine and boring, they also help us order our lives and get things done.

So if you're serious about running, the best way to make sure it gets done is to make it part of your routine. Having a set time to run—every morning, every other evening after work, during lunch hours, or something similar—makes running a regular activity, a habit. A routine is especially important when working toward a specific goal, as in training for a race.

Spiritual routines are important too. In Acts, we learn this about the early church:

All the believers devoted themselves to the apostles' teaching, and to fellowship, and to sharing in meals (including the Lord's Supper), and to prayer. (Acts 2:42)

All the believers were meeting regularly at the Temple in the area known as Solomon's Colonnade. (Acts 5:12)

Everyone was "devoted" to each other, to prayer, and to learning from God's Word. And they met "regularly." In other words, they had a routine, a schedule that worked for them.

The Runner

Jen thought she should take up running to lose a few pounds and to keep in shape. So she found the running trail in a nearby forest preserve, got advice from friends who were avid runners, and bought a running outfit and a good pair of shoes. She decided to begin on Saturday, and she was able to run/walk a mile. Encouraged, she ran again on Sunday afternoon. She had to get to the office early Monday, and Tuesday was jammed, so she wasn't able to even think about running until Wednesday—but the rain kept her inside. Over the next couple of months, she ran only a few times.

When Rico decided to train for a half marathon, he knew he would have to keep a running schedule—more than his occasional neighborhood jogs. So he made a commitment to get up an hour early and run first thing every day, rain or shine, making sure that he had the right gear for rain and cooler weather. He reserved Saturdays for his longer runs and used Sunday as a day to rest and recover. Rico stuck to his schedule and had a great race.

Bodie had always been in sports, so he was used to working out on a regular basis. When he began running in his thirties, he had no trouble inserting a time to run in his daily schedule. As a relatively new Christian, Bodie had become involved in a church and a fellowship group. In one of their meetings, the discussion focused on personal spiritual growth and the importance of having regular times of Bible study and prayer. Bodie decided to go that way, and he knew exactly what to do. Taking the same approach that he had for running, he put thirty minutes in his daily schedule for reading a passage of Scripture, answering questions about it, and praying.

The Race

Sometimes our spiritual exercises and experiences can become routine in the wrong way. That is, we can simply go through the motions at worship, Bible study, and even prayer. Jesus spoke against meaningless rituals: "When you pray, don't babble on and on as people of other religions do. They think their prayers are answered merely by repeating their words again and again" (Matthew 6:7). But the answer isn't to be unscheduled or unorganized. If we take that route, we may not study, pray, or worship for meaningful stretches of time as other activities and responsibilities fill up our schedules . . . or we may just forget.

The Result

From prison, in what would be his last residence on earth, Paul wrote these words to Timothy: "Run from anything that stimulates youthful lusts. Instead, pursue righteous living, faithfulness, love, and peace. Enjoy the companionship of those who call on the Lord with pure hearts" (2 Timothy 2:22).

Timothy was a "professional"; that is, he was a pastor, someone engaged in full-time Christian ministry. Paul knew that spiritual practices could have become commonplace and monotonous. So he encouraged Timothy to "run" and to "pursue" the kind of life God wanted him to live.

Don't take your relationship with God for granted. Make matters of faith your pursuit, establishing a regular routine of spiritual disciplines.

My Story

I had disciplined myself to run every evening—and I was doing it! But then I decided to make my daily run a spiritual experience. Usually that wasn't the case—far from it. At times I would wear headphones and listen to the news or a game. Sometimes I'd run with my iPod and listen to my favorite running music—you know, the kind with the energetic beat—very motivational. I'd also wear the GPS and regularly check my pace and distance.

Yes, I know that a "spiritual experience" can be different for different people, but I felt convicted about not praying enough, so I decided to pray while I ran, with no earphones or other distractions on me. To do that, I carefully measured the distance of each of the neighborhood running routes I usually took. Then before leaving the house, I decided how many miles to run and chose the appropriate route. And I wrote down my leaving time and checked the clock at the end of each run to see if I needed to pick up my pace the next time. I also wrote prayer requests on a card that I could carry. Those steps helped me focus on praying . . . all the way. And they provided a way for me to "pursue" a godly life.

Jermaine

Think It Through

1. Where does worship fit into your schedule? How about fellowship with other believers?
2. How and when do you have regular teaching from the Bible?
3. When would you like to have a daily time of Bible reading and prayer?
4. What can you do to establish a more spiritually productive routine?

On Running

How can I keep from getting fatigued?

You can take a few simple steps to reduce fatigue. The first is through efficient movement. Some runners, for example, waste a lot of energy simply by allowing their arms to almost flail as they run. The more efficient your movement, the less you will become fatigued. Spend time on your technique. Practice makes permanent; only *perfect* practice makes perfect. So focus on your stride length, rate, and so forth. Second, you can double your energy stores (the fuel for your muscles) through training well and eating well. Finally, you need to know yourself and your ability. Yes, you should push yourself in training, but pushing too hard or too quickly will cause you to tire sooner.

JOURNAL

_____

_____

_____

_____

_____

_____

_____

_____

_____

_____

_____

_____

_____

RUNNING LOG

	TIME	DISTANCE	WEATHER	NOTES
DAY 1				
DAY 2				
DAY 3				
DAY 4				
DAY 5				

ESTABLISH A ROUTINE

Those who have made running a part of their daily or weekly schedule are often able to carry that discipline into other areas of life, even the spiritual. They may, for example, establish a regular time of intense, personal prayer.

Daniel may be the best biblical example of someone who had established a spiritual routine. As a young man in Babylon, where he had been taken as a captive after Judah's defeat, he could have succumbed to frustration and despair, or he could have given in to the pressures of the culture and tried to fit in, to be like the pagans around him. Instead, he remained faithful to God and continued his practice of daily prayer, even after a law had been signed that required everyone to worship an idol. "When Daniel learned that the law had been signed, he went home and knelt down as usual in his upstairs room, with its windows open toward Jerusalem. He prayed three times a day, just as he had always done, giving thanks to his God" (Daniel 6:10).

Two points jump out in this passage. First, Daniel knelt in prayer "as usual"; this was his daily practice. Second, Daniel prayed with the "windows open"; he didn't hide his devotion to God. Daniel was able to remain strong in his faith and faithful to his commitment to God because of the focus of his life and his continual communication with the Father.

The Runner

The book of Daniel begins with this story:

> *The king ordered Ashpenaz, his chief of staff, to bring to the palace some of the young men of Judah's royal family and other noble families, who had been brought to Babylon as captives. "Select only strong, healthy, and good-looking young men," he said. "Make sure they are well versed in every branch of learning, are gifted with knowledge and good judgment, and are suited to serve in the royal palace. Train these young men in the language and literature of Babylon." The king assigned them a daily ration of food and wine from his own kitchens. They were to be trained for three years, and then they would enter the royal service.*
> (DANIEL 1:3-5)

These young men were selected for an elite training program in the kingdom. But Daniel and three of his friends didn't go along with the *whole* program. They were selective about their diet, insisting on eating vegetables instead of the king's rich food. And they proposed a ten-day test to see who would be in better shape. "At the end of the ten days, Daniel and his three friends looked healthier and better nourished than the young men who had been eating the food assigned by the king. So after that, the attendant fed them only vegetables instead of the food and wine provided for the others" (Daniel 1:15-16).

These men were disciplined in all areas. We don't know their exercise routine, but we can imagine the four of them rising early and running a prescribed course around the great city of Babylon. They wanted to be physically and spiritually healthy—to honor God.

The Race

Those involved in organized sports often explain that the experience of working out, practicing, and developing skills and stamina teaches them how to use their time well and to be disciplined. No one has more time than anyone else; we all get twenty-four hours a day. But some people accomplish more during their allotted hours because they know how to establish a routine and then keep to it. This certainly is true with running. Face it, on some mornings (or evenings) we can feel totally unmotivated to pull on those shoes and get going. We may not feel well, or the weather might be cold, wet, humid, hot, or windy. We can always find an excuse if we try. But disciplined runners go out anyway. Some runners find others to join them so they can encourage each other.

Spiritual "runners" need to take the same approach in their relationship with God. The writer of Psalm 119 declares, "I will pursue your commands, for you expand my understanding" (Psalm 119:32). This statement implies an intentional effort to continually understand God's Word and then do what it says. Regular—daily—routine.

The Result

Regular communication is basic to any strong relationship with anyone, God included. And the great news is that he wants to speak and listen to us. Communication with God comes mainly through his written Word and prayer. As we read and study the Bible, we learn about God and his will—principles for living. Regular time in God's Word is imperative.

So is prayer. Yes, we can (and should) talk with God throughout the day—before meals, in moments of decision or stress, and in times of gratitude and praise. But we also need concentrated times of in-depth conversation, when we pour out our feelings and requests or simply sit in silence, contemplating God's goodness and thanking him for who he is and what he has done.

These habits need to be part of our daily routine.

My Story

Usually whatever I am studying or working on in my
Christian life somehow makes it into my running life.
One of the more memorable examples occurred several
years ago when I was training for a spring marathon
while simultaneously doing a study on spiritual
disciplines. I was learning that spiritual disciplines
allow us to become the people we want to be. When we
respond in a way that is un-Christlike—whether that's
inappropriately expressed anger, bitterness, jealousy,
or something else—we are simply expressing outwardly
what is in our hearts. If we want to change the result
on the outside, we must consistently practice spiritual
disciplines to change our hearts inside first. This was
the focus of my Bible study as we headed into the dark
Chicago winter.

I have always considered the time between Labor Day
and Christmas to be the "golden time" for running in
Chicago. With the worst of the heat and humidity gone,
despite some cold November winds, you can generally
find good running weather most weeks at that time
of year.

After Christmas, however, the situation changes
quickly. Snow and ice are constant threats, and the
already-cold temperatures drop another ten degrees
or so, just enough to make it difficult to assemble
sufficient layers to stay warm.

Because I was scheduled to run an early-April
marathon, my peak training weeks fell to February,
a dicey proposition. This winter proved especially
difficult even by Chicago standards, with lots of snow
in January. So I was forced to cut a lot of my runs
short due to cold or ice and snow on the roads. My
hope was that I would increase my mileage in February
to make sure I had a sufficient base to tackle the
marathon. Unfortunately, February proved even worse

than January for getting outside. I ended up cutting out at least one run per week, and my long runs went from a planned eighteen to twenty miles to ten to fifteen. The longest run I was able to get in the entire winter was sixteen miles. Still, I remained optimistic that my previous training would help, and because I had several marathons under my belt at that point, I felt I could make it through anything race day would throw at me.

On race day, knowing that my training was not all it could have been, I started the race at an easier pace than I normally would have. The idea was to go slow to ensure I had plenty of energy left for the late miles. The early miles were uneventful, but I noticed around the halfway point that I was not feeling as fresh as I normally did. From there a section of the course heads downhill for a while, but at around mile sixteen the course gradually goes uphill. As soon as I saw the hill at mile sixteen, I knew I was in trouble. By mile eighteen I had thrown out all hopes of keeping my (seemingly easy) pace intact for the entire race. By mile twenty I had slowed another minute per mile in my pace, and around mile twenty-three it was all over.

As I began my three- or four-mile "death march" (the phrase I used when talking to myself during the race) to the finish line, I thought of my lack of training: the long runs cut short, the base miles not run early in the winter, the complete lack of "tempo" runs to keep up my cardiovascular endurance. What did I expect to happen on race day?

Through my discomfort and anguish as I sheepishly ran the last quarter mile (to keep up appearances, of course), I thought, *Ah, yes, and what do you expect to happen in your life when you cut short things like giving sacrificially, your prayer time, your time studying the Word, etc.? Yep, a death march.*

Mike

Think It Through

1. What keeps you from developing spiritual routines?
2. When would be the best time each day for you to read your Bible and pray?
3. Devotional books like this one can help. What other resources do you need for your daily routine?
4. Which friend(s) could you enlist to encourage you and hold you accountable?

On Running

What are some principles of goal setting?

The most important principle of goal setting is to write down your goals. You can't monitor them if they aren't written down. Set specific goals—what you want to accomplish and when. Set difficult but realistic goals. Set short-term goals to reach long-term ones (*very* important in marathon running). Think all the way through the process, setting outcome, performance, and progress goals. If you're racing, set goals for training as well as for the race. Record how and what you're doing. Be sure to consider your own personality and motivations, and find a support system for reaching your goals. Finally, find someone else to provide an evaluation and give you feedback.

JOURNAL

_____

_____

_____

_____

_____

_____

RUNNING LOG

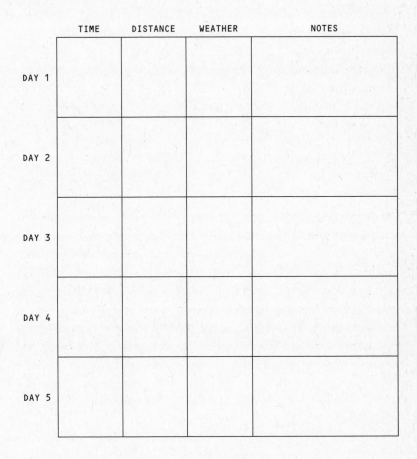

	TIME	DISTANCE	WEATHER	NOTES
DAY 1				
DAY 2				
DAY 3				
DAY 4				
DAY 5				

JUST DO IT

Let's face it—sometimes we just don't feel like running. And our lack of motivation might not be just physical. We could be dealing with a relational conflict, financial stress, or demands at work, or every hour of the week could suddenly seem filled with appointments and obligations.

At other times, threatening weather conditions could cause us to pause as we consider heading out for a run. We know the pain and frustration of running in severe cold or hot temps or through rain or heavy humidity.

In all these situations, one of the easiest responses is to skip the run that day . . . or week. We may be able to get away with missing a workout for a day if our schedule includes daily jaunts. But if we run every other day and miss one, we end up with three days between runs. Even worse, we can develop the habit of finding excuses for not running and soon lose our routine.

Paul knew that the believers in the city of Colosse were in danger of losing their spiritual motivation. Being identified with Christ in that culture could bring alienation and persecution. Believers needed courage to press on, to consistently practice their faith. So Paul encouraged these men and women and prayed for them, that they would have "endurance and patience":

> *We have not stopped praying for you since we first heard about*
> *you. We ask God to give you complete knowledge of his will and*
> *to give you spiritual wisdom and understanding. Then the way*
> *you live will always honor and please the Lord, and your lives*
> *will produce every kind of good fruit. All the while, you will grow*
> *as you learn to know God better and better.*
>
> *We also pray that you will be strengthened with all his*
> *glorious power so you will have all the endurance and patience*
> *you need. May you be filled with joy, always thanking the Father.*
>
> (COLOSSIANS 1:9-12)

The Runner

"Spiritual disciplines"—she had heard that expression several times and had decided to see what it meant. So she picked up a recommended book and dug in. Soon she felt convicted about her lack of certain internal spiritual practices and decided she needed to schedule daily prayer and Bible study and regular times of silence and solitude. The best time of day seemed to be the evening, just after she put the kids to bed. So she found a quiet place in the house and put her Bible, notebook, and devotional resources on the table.

The first couple of days went well. She had no problem winding down from the day and spending quality time with God. Occasionally the times would be interrupted by a phone call she felt she had to take. And every now and then she would finish some housework, reasoning that if she didn't do it then, it wouldn't get done. Those breaks in the schedule meant that her focused time with God became more sporadic than regular. Then, when a couple of her favorite TV shows aired in that time slot, she dropped the practice altogether.

The Race

Our "runner" had allowed small issues to crowd out her spiritual practice, the insignificant to replace the important. She needed a dose of "endurance and patience," the courage to "just do it!" regardless of pressing issues or swirling circumstances.

Excuse making comes easy, especially when it means avoiding a difficult or demanding task. We can always find a "reason" *not* to run, and in the case of spiritual disciplines, we also have the devil whispering the excuses: "You're too tired." "You deserve a break." "Do it tomorrow." "You've done enough for this week." "You can pray as you fall asleep."

Once we give in and break our routine, we abandon our positive habit and develop the new habit of making excuses.

The Result

You know what happens when you haven't run in a while—you get out of shape. In fact, before long you can feel sluggish and may even begin to add a few unwanted pounds. To stay in shape spiritually, we need regular "workouts" where we exercise our faith and nourish our souls. You have a plan and you've built a routine—make no excuses.

"My dear brothers and sisters, be strong and immovable. Always work enthusiastically for the Lord, for you know that nothing you do for the Lord is ever useless" (1 Corinthians 15:58).

Just do it!

My Story

"Mary, lift those knees up! . . . Don't look down; look up and all around you. . . . Pick your feet up. I can hear you shuffling."

Ugh . . . these are just some of the things my coach reminds me to do every time we're out running. Some things you need to know about my coach: He's faster than me; he's an athletic nut; he's my best friend; he's my husband. His motto: Running cures everything.

"Just run," he says.

"I have a cold."

"No problem. Running will cure you."

"I have a headache."

"You will feel better after a quick run."

And you know what? He's right, because after a "quick run" you'll have other aches and pains that take your mind off of the original ailment!

Another of my husband's mottos: No man, woman, or dog gets left behind. Yes, dog. We run with our two dogs. I trail behind all three . . . because I'm the poop patrol.

One other motto that my husband believes: You can do it. In rain, in sleet, in freezing temperatures, and in ninety-degree heat. Put your mind to it, and just do it.

All of my husband's mottos are examples of God in my life: Just pray!—God is always listening. Just run!— he will cure everything that ails you. No one gets left behind!—God will never leave you, no matter what. Lastly, just do it!—live your life fully relying on God because he has a plan for each and every one of us.

Mary

Think It Through

1. What types of issues and interruptions often tempt you to suspend your running routine? What helps you keep to your schedule?

2. What challenges did you have to overcome to establish your spiritual routines?

3. Which of these spiritual practices are you most likely to rationalize skipping: worship, service, Bible study, prayer, silence and solitude, evangelism? What excuses do you use?

4. What can you do to be more disciplined in your pursuit of knowing God's will, spiritual wisdom, and understanding (Colossians 1:9)?

On Running

How should I eat?

Your eating proportions may be different from other runners. Your calorie intake should be in this proportion: 55–60 percent from carbohydrates, 25–30 percent from fat (one-third from saturated fat), and the remainder from protein. One way to figure out the amount of protein is to have 1–1.6 grams of protein per kilogram of body weight. And of course, always find ways to drink plenty of fluids.

JOURNAL

_____

_____

_____

_____

_____

_____

_____

_____

_____

_____

_____

_____

_____

_____

_____

_____

_____

_____

RUNNING LOG

	TIME	DISTANCE	WEATHER	NOTES
DAY 1				
DAY 2				
DAY 3				
DAY 4				
DAY 5				

JUST DO IT

Check out this verse: "They will not get tired or stumble. They will not stop for rest or sleep. Not a belt will be loose, not a sandal strap broken" (Isaiah 5:27). Now that's the way to run a race!

Actually, this is a prophecy about God's punishment on those who "have rejected the law of the LORD of Heaven's Armies . . . [and] have despised the word of the Holy One of Israel" (Isaiah 5:24). God promised to empower these invaders to execute his judgment. But the point is that God would enable these soldiers to run successfully, without rest and with no equipment failures, to do his work. On their own, the invaders would never be able to complete that course.

God wants to empower us to do his will. That's why Paul told the believers in Philippi, "God is working in you, giving you the desire and the power to do what pleases him" (Philippians 2:13). Later he declared, "I can do everything through Christ, who gives me strength" (Philippians 4:13).

We should be relentless, determined to do what we know God wants us to do.

The Runner

"Come on—get going—pick it up," the coach yelled as his runners circled the track. Travis was bone tired, his lungs bursting, and the rain was stinging his face, but he pushed through. Finally there was a break to grab some water, catch his breath, and stretch a bit. But Travis knew the rest would be short; soon the whistle would blow and they'd circle the track four more times . . . another mile.

What's wrong with that man? thought Travis. *Coach is an animal— he needs to get out here and do this; he probably wouldn't make a lap.* The thought brought a smile to his face. *He's killing us out here—it's getting dark; the wind is picking up; the rain is getting stronger; the track is slippery; I'm at my limit. . . .*

Then, almost as if he were reading Travis's mind, Coach said, "Look, guys. I know you're tired and these are miserable conditions. But the only way for us to be successful in this sport is to put in the miles, to work hard, no matter what. We don't know what the weather will be like at the meets. But if we can run in this, we'll be ready for anything! Remember our goal—to win state! Now let's get going!" And off they ran again.

The Race

Travis had a coach to train, encourage, motivate, and push him through the hard times. And his coach would accept no excuses. Rain or shine, they ran.

While we're living for Christ, at times the course can seem impossible, the conditions terrible, and the obstacles insurmountable. We can be tempted to give up. Excuses can flow quickly through our minds. We can think, *Are you kidding? I can't go on. I don't have the strength or the endurance!*

We'd be right, of course. But God doesn't intend for us to live the Christian life on our own. He empowers us "to do what pleases him." God is not only a "coach" who prods us along through his Word; he's also an inner resource, giving us the desire and the power to follow him.

The Result

If you don't know what God wants, ask him to tell you, to show you in his Word. If you know what he wants you to do, just do it . . . depending on him and in his power. Remember, "despite all these things, overwhelming victory is ours through Christ, who loved us" (Romans 8:37).

My Story

As a runner, if I had a dollar for every time I've told myself to "just do it," I would be rich! Training for a marathon is a long and grueling process that requires at least eighteen weeks of running five days a week, building up your mileage to about fifty miles per week. That is a lot of pounding the pavement, oftentimes running the same route over and over again, step after step after step—pretty boring at times, that's for sure! On many mornings (usually the cold, dark, rainy ones), I would much rather stay in bed. And I have those times when I start my run only to realize my body is not cooperating and is just plain tired. Oh, how I would love to just cut the run short or stop entirely! But I can't. That voice in my head keeps saying, *Just do it! No excuses. Be tough and get out there and run.*

I've learned with both running and life that we can make excuses to quit or to *not* do something very easy. No one will really care. No one may even know. But the courage and strength it takes to "just do it" even when no one else does, or cares, are what build our bodies to be able to complete that 10K or marathon, and they build our character to help us become the people God wants us to be. It's not easy, but God never promised that life would be easy. And he does promise that our work for him will not be in vain. He will not leave us or forsake us and will be with us every step of the way—step after step after step after step.

Ellen

Think It Through

1. When have you felt totally unmotivated while preparing to run? What happened? What made you decide to put on those shoes and get after it?
2. When have you felt totally unmotivated in your life of faith? Do you know what caused your lack of motivation?
3. What obstacles and issues have you found most difficult to deal with in the Christian life? Where did you find the motivation and strength to tackle them?
4. What can you do to rely more completely on God's strength working in and through you?

On Running

How can I mentally prepare for my next running workout?

When getting ready for a workout, try to concentrate completely on that event, blocking out irrelevant thoughts and focusing on what is controllable. Mentally rehearse your workout—course, leg stride, rhythm, etc. Have a detailed plan for your run, considering how your body responds to different stimuli (for example, what causes anxiety or another response). Be ready for those anticipated situations, or strategize ways to avoid them.

JOURNAL

RUNNING LOG

	TIME	DISTANCE	WEATHER	NOTES
DAY 1				
DAY 2				
DAY 3				
DAY 4				
DAY 5				

WARM UP

Can't wait—in a hurry—gotta get going—get this over with—only so much time. . . .

Thoughts like these push us out the door to get the workout in, and then we are on our way. "Run and done" is our motto. We do that to our peril, risking pulled muscles and more.

Serious athletes in all sports know the importance of warming up before a contest in order to prepare their muscles, joints, ligaments, and other body parts for the strain that will be placed on them. If you get to the stadium or field beforehand, you'll see a lot of jogging and stretching, pulling and pushing on the muscles and ligaments about to be used. These athletes want to do their best; they also want to avoid injury. In running, many injuries occur because the runners fail to stretch or prepare the body in other ways.

All of this speaks to being properly prepared for the run, for the race, and for life. Rushing through a quiet time with the Lord or rushing into spiritual service may hurt us much more than a pulled muscle.

Centuries ago, Solomon wrote, "Too much activity gives you restless dreams; too many words make you a fool" (Ecclesiastes 5:3). True enough. In the case of running, he could have added, "Too much activity *too soon*."

The Runner

He was ready, having carefully followed the marathon workout schedule for the past couple of months. He knew his endurance was increasing; he didn't begin to break a sweat until almost five miles. And he actually looked forward to the long run of the week, especially if the weather conditions were right. Just a few weeks to go before the big race!

But his day was crazy at work, and his afternoon meeting went on *forever*! Then he drove into a traffic snag that doubled his drive time. So as he pulled into the driveway, he was frustrated and couldn't wait to get out of his suit and into his jogging outfit and run. Literally, he couldn't wait. So he didn't stretch at all—just started running. And because he had started late, he began much faster than normal.

Just a couple of miles in, he felt his left hamstring tighten, but he kept running . . . until the pain almost knocked him to the ground.

The run had ended . . . as had his marathon dreams.

The Race

In the early days of the church, the apostle Paul wrote these instructions to Timothy, his young pastor protégé: "Never be in a hurry about appointing a church leader" (1 Timothy 5:22). Paul was seeking to protect the church from immature leadership that might lead to failure. Instead he said that Timothy should make sure that leaders in the church were mature believers, with theological knowledge, a solid reputation, and a track record of positive, moral living. In his hurry to establish the church, Timothy might have been tempted to appoint, install, or ordain young believers who looked and sounded good but weren't adequately grounded in the faith.

We run the same risk today when we ask new Christians to lead Bible studies or elect them to positions of responsibility in the church.

We do it with young people by holding them up as examples of mature Christians (they often fall off that pedestal). We do it when we act as if we have all the answers when, in fact, we harbor serious doubts.

Even if we're not quite ready for leadership, it shouldn't discourage us from working in the church or serving God in other ministries. Regardless of how long we've been following Jesus, we should be careful about jumping into leadership without adequate preparation—we don't want to pull a spiritual muscle.

Some things shouldn't be rushed.

The Result

As a committed follower of Christ, you want to serve him . . . and you should. But be careful about taking on more than you can handle, considering your level of spiritual maturity and life experience. You wouldn't ask a high school student for marriage advice. You wouldn't ask a private to lead you into battle. You wouldn't hire a recent college graduate to manage a professional baseball team. And if you were that student, private, or recent grad, although you would be flattered by any of those opportunities, you would be foolish to accept them. Each one would be a recipe for disaster. Some things shouldn't be rushed. Take time to warm up and stretch before hitting your stride.

My Story

At 5:00 a.m., the guesthouse doors are still locked, but a quiet exit out the window and a quick shinny down the corner post of the front porch roof makes that a nonissue. The chickens and a cat who doesn't want to be seen are awake, but no one else is. The city is oddly quiet in the predawn glow coming from the water. I know this is going to be one of those runs, an experience that takes me somewhere only runners can comprehend. Despite my desire to sprint, I start out with restraint.

Each November, the tiny Chinese territory of Macau is transformed into the hub of Formula racing as it hosts the Macau Grand Prix. One of the most challenging auto-racing courses in the world is assembled on the edge of the South China Sea, tucked along the waterfront, and threaded up the subtle hillsides. The course is one of the narrowest to be raced anywhere. A tight 180-degree turn called the Melco Hairpin squeezes the course down to just twenty-two feet. During the rest of the year, it's not difficult to find the red-and-yellow striping painted on curbs, corners, and permanent barricades. I plan to run as much of the course as possible.

Finding my way out of the neighborhood is easy. The water provides a point of reference from just about anywhere within the territory. The challenge is finding the *right* water. A few hundred years ago, Macau was an island, but a pair of sandbars on the north end joined, and the tiny territory now has twenty-five miles of coast and two-tenths of a mile connecting it to Guangdong Province in China.

Nevertheless, the "major water" of the expansive China Sea serves as my guide to the Formula racing circuit. The start and finish of the course is surrounded by water with the section leading up to it on a narrow breakwater that protects a reservoir.

A steady ten minutes at an easy pace, and suddenly I see the red-and-white striping crisscrossed with telltale tire skids, silently telling stories of very loud events.

I fall into a rhythm on the course and am struck by the aromas. Macau has the highest population density on the planet. The half million residents squeeze into eleven square miles—forty-five thousand folks for every square mile. So this is an urban adventure. And with so many mouths to feed, breakfast starts early.

The smell of chicken eases out of an apartment complex to my right as I work my way through the Solitude Esses. Odd choice for breakfast, but then again, it could be something that simply tastes like chicken. A flowering

shrub clings to its small section of wall, launching a
sweet fragrance into the morning. After that a musty smell
floats up from a small water run-off that passes under the
road—then a spice of some kind, almost like paprika.

Lisboa Bend introduces a straight section, levels
out, and provides views of the harbor. Right about now
I realize that I may be running opposite the direction
the circuit is raced. Oh well—makes my experience more
unique, I guess.

Down toward the harbor and casinos, there is still an
eerie lack of activity for a city so full of people. It's
peaceful.

Then it hits me. I'm on a racing circuit where millions
of dollars are spent on going fast, and I'm thoroughly
enjoying traveling eight miles an hour. I see life, my
life. The total tonnage of what I miss out on while
ripping through life at Mach 1 flashes before me. And
running appears once again as a gift.

Ironic. I'm running, but in doing so, I'm slowing down
and taking in the nuances. I'm experiencing things others
miss. I've come to believe, and have proven time and
again, that the best way to experience someplace new is
to go there and run. In this primitive activity performed
by humans since creation, we push aside the filters modern
life surrounds us with and settle into the essential. We
learn, we smell, we feel, we live.

Todd

Think It Through

1. When have you seen a young or inexperienced person thrust into a
   leadership role prematurely? What happened?
2. In what ways might we be tempted to rush spiritual maturity? Why is
   that tendency problematic?
3. What does "warming up" spiritually mean to you? How will that help
   you in the long run?

On Running

How important is flexibility to running well?

Flexibility increases the elasticity of the connective tissue and muscles and decreases injuries. Stretching and flexibility training will increase your range of motion and alleviate muscle and joint pain. The more flexible your muscles are, the better your running stride and efficiency will be. Tight muscles can shorten your stride, making you work harder and tire sooner.

JOURNAL

_____

_____

_____

_____

_____

RUNNING LOG

	TIME	DISTANCE	WEATHER	NOTES
DAY 1				
DAY 2				
DAY 3				
DAY 4				
DAY 5				

WARM UP

Another reason some runners fail to warm up properly is a macho attitude. Confident in their athletic ability and eager to get going (and feeling young and fit), they rush out and on their way. That approach may work for some for a while, but the possible problems are not worth the risk. This proverb, a warning for all areas of life, should cause us to think twice about preparing adequately: "Pride goes before destruction, and haughtiness before a fall" (Proverbs 16:18).

As finite and frail human beings, we need to recognize our weaknesses and prepare accordingly. Failing to do so would be foolish indeed.

We're also vulnerable in other areas, and in this sinful world, we're surrounded by temptations. Again, to not recognize this fact and take precautions could be disastrous. The apostle Paul warns, "If you think you are standing strong, be careful not to fall" (1 Corinthians 10:12).

The Runner

We know from news reports and from personal experience about the moral failings of those who did not heed those warnings:

- the financial adviser who used money from new clients to cover losses from previous poor investments and slipped into a Ponzi scheme
- the charity worker who "borrowed" a little from the donations till, but that "just once" became a habit
- the employee's innocuous flirtations with a coworker that turned into an affair
- the addict who began by "experimenting" with drugs
- the pastor who became attracted to a counselee

These life-runners pulled up lame because they thought they were immune and because they hadn't taken preventative precautions. And in the process, they ignored the warning signs and rushed by the opportunities to get back on course.

The Race

Being prepared for temptations ("warming up" for that challenge) means thinking through the possibilities and how we should respond in various tempting situations. For example, we may think through scenarios like these:

- "If I'm asked to do _____, then I will respond by saying _____ and doing _____."
- "If this happens, then I will react this way."

And so forth. And we certainly should avoid situations where we're pretty sure we'll be tempted. Being prepared also means putting up safeguards, barriers to ensure that we won't cross into forbidden territory.

In all of this we should realize that we can't resist in our strength alone, so we should ask God for his wisdom and strength to resist. Listen to this powerful passage that comes right after the verse we looked at earlier: "The temptations in your life are no different from what others experience. And God is faithful. He will not allow the temptation to be more than you can stand. When you are tempted, he will show you a way out so that you can endure" (1 Corinthians 10:13).

The Result

Regardless of our precautions, we can't avoid all temptations. That would be like assuming we will never have leg or joint problems or encounter animals, cars, and potholes when we run. But did you catch God's promises in that passage? He said he will not allow you to be tempted "more than you can stand" and that he will provide a way of escape. So here's a suggestion: When you're tempted to take a wrong turn in life, pray and say something like this: "Thank you, Lord, for trusting me that much! Now, what do you want me to do?" Then look for his way of escape and take it.

My Story

"My steps have stayed on your path; I have not wavered from following you" (Psalm 17:5).

At mile seventeen, I didn't think I was going to do it. I had turned my right ankle twice, once trying to negotiate a construction cone at mile four and again in a hole on the trail at mile eight. Despite this, I managed to continue moving my feet, which felt like lead by mile fifteen.

When I ran through the ballooned arch at the finish, I fully realized I had done it. For the first time in my life I had run twenty miles. But following the shock and exhilaration of "I made it" came conviction. The Lord let me know in very clear terms that I had failed to invite him into *every* step of the run. Yes, I had prayed the "Oh God, help me" kind of prayer, but I had not involved him on the "step-by-step" level. He wants to be there, step by step, in every "run" of my life.

I need to deliberately consider him, thank him, trust him, and recognize him at each and *every* step of the way.

Twenty miles is a long way to run on one's own strength and energy. Yet I try to live that way in many areas of life. Instead, I need to involve God in each and every step.

My next training run was twenty-three miles, and he was right there, step by step.

Cheryl

Think It Through

1. When have you recently seen overconfidence contribute to a favored athlete or team losing a contest?
2. When has pride preceded a fall for you?
3. What are your most common and most pressing temptations?
4. What precautions have you taken to avoid them? What ways of escape has God given you?

On Running

How do I prepare to run in the heat?

The best way to prepare to run in any kind of weather, especially heat, is to become acclimated to it. That means spending time in that weather, preferably five to ten days with heat. After a few days, your body will start to sweat sooner and distribute sweat better. Your sweat will also be more diluted. So don't try running long distances at your normal pace the first day in hot weather. Allow your body to become used to the weather first.

JOURNAL

_____

_____

_____

_____

_____

RUNNING LOG

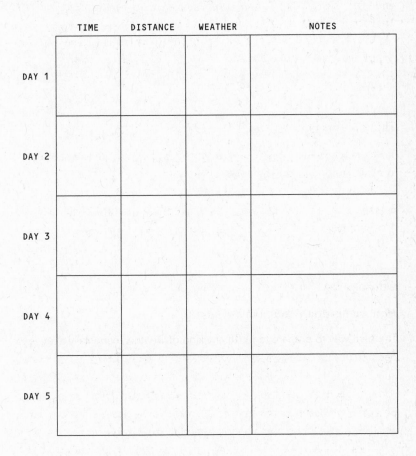

	TIME	DISTANCE	WEATHER	NOTES
DAY 1				
DAY 2				
DAY 3				
DAY 4				
DAY 5				

DEAL WITH IT

Overcoming inertia, lacing up the shoes, opening the door, and putting one foot in front of the other, regardless of our great excuses to *not* run, is commendable—and should be the norm. At times, however, we'll encounter issues that must be dealt with. Usually these are physical symptoms that could signal severe problems down the road. It could be a hot spot on a foot, a weakness in a knee, or a pain in the back, ankle, or Achilles tendon. We would be foolish to ignore those warning signs and try to run through them. Instead, we should listen to our bodies and take corrective and healing action instead of making the situation worse.

Spiritual warning signs appear as well, and we ignore them to our peril. The signs can include feeling pulled toward a persistent temptation, developing a critical spirit, becoming apathetic about worship and personal Bible study, falling into old habits, losing hope and joy, and others. When we sense any of these warnings, we need to deal with them immediately and take corrective action. That means turning to the Great Physician. That's what David did, and here's what happened: "O LORD my God, I cried to you for help, and you restored my health" (Psalm 30:2).

Later he wrote this: "He heals the brokenhearted and bandages their wounds" (Psalm 147:3).

The Runner

Right at the last mile he felt a twinge in his right knee, just after stepping in the small pothole in the street. "That'll teach me to run in the dark," he muttered. He didn't think much of the incident, figuring he'd run through it . . . and he did.

But the next evening at the beginning of his run, he felt pain in that knee—not debilitating, but noticeable. He stopped and stretched, then started up again. The pain didn't subside, but it didn't get worse, so he continued and finished five miles. On his next run, the pain was there and felt about the same, so he kept going but favored the sore leg a bit. The following morning, his left ankle was sore, and he still felt the pain in his right knee. That evening he debated about running, considering how his legs were feeling, but he had a schedule he needed to keep to be in shape for the race . . . so he ran again. Halfway through, shooting pain in his knee stopped him in his tracks, and he limped home.

Soon the orthopedic doctor confirmed what he had feared: a torn meniscus. He needed arthroscopic surgery and wouldn't be running for a while. His doctor said, "I'm glad you came when you did. Any more running would have risked much greater damage. You wouldn't believe what I've seen here, with runners who won't stop until the pain becomes unbearable. Discipline is one thing, but that's just stupid!"

The Race

As is the case with many dedicated runners, we can become so busy with our daily routines and jammed schedules that we ignore or run through our spiritual twinges of pain—warning signs that something might be wrong. Most drivers, when they see "check engine" or "check oil" lights flash on the dashboard, have the car serviced as soon as possible. They don't want to risk serious engine damage. The same can happen in our relationship with God. When the warning light comes on, we can choose to ignore it or get help. John writes, "If we claim we have no sin, we are only fooling ourselves and not living in the truth" (1 John 1:8). In other words, if we pretend we don't have a problem, we're foolish and headed for trouble.

The warning could be the twinge of conscience that makes us feel guilty about something we've thought or done. It might be the convicting nudge of the Holy Spirit during a worship service. It could be a Christian friend confronting us about a poor choice, a sinful action, or a misplaced priority. Usually the corrective process begins with confession, admitting our weakness and sin to our loving heavenly Father. John continues with this great promise: "If we confess our sins to him, he is faithful and just to forgive us our sins and to cleanse us from all wickedness" (1 John 1:9).

The Result

Just as with going to the doctor, confession is the beginning. Sometimes surgery will be necessary as God begins changing your attitudes and desires. You may have to work on a relationship issue if another person is involved. The prescription may mean canceling subscriptions or finding new friends or places to hang out. Whatever God is telling you through that warning sign, you need to deal with it.

And here's another psalm to remember: "The LORD helps the fallen and lifts those bent beneath their loads" (Psalm 145:14). Run with that promise!

My Story

I had decided to run a marathon—a huge challenge for me, a big guy and a non-runner. But I found a sixteen-week training schedule and stuck to it. The twenty-mile run came at the end of the twelfth week. It was tough, but I made it with the help of a friend from church. After that

I knew I could finish the marathon. Worst-case scenario,
I would run 20 miles and then walk or crawl my way through
the last 6.2. Either way, I would have accomplished
my goal.

Several days later I went out to run a few miles, but
after a block, shooting pains in my foot almost knocked
me down. I stretched the foot, walked a block, and then
tried to run again. The pain returned. Thinking it was
just soreness from the long run, I rested a few days. When
I tried again, the pain returned, and my confidence turned
to worry. Not only would I not be able to finish the
race, in this condition I wouldn't be able to even start.
The doctor diagnosed the problem as plantar fasciitis
and recommended that I stay off my feet because the foot
needed rest to heal.

I followed the doctor's orders and didn't run at all.
Then I tried to run a week prior to the race, but I still
felt some pain. So I realized that my chance of running
the marathon was a long shot. During this time I prayed a
lot, not in bitterness but to say that I felt like I was
on a journey and that I would welcome wherever God was
sending me in this trial.

Later that week, some experienced runners suggested I
try a different pair of shoes to see if that might help.
It was worth a shot. So I went to a specialty running
store on the Thursday before the Sunday marathon and
bought a pair of shoes they recommended. I decided I would
let my foot rest until Saturday; then, if I could run the
three-mile loop in my subdivision without pain, I would
try running on Sunday.

That Saturday, I remember thinking only a miracle could
make my foot pain-free. After the first few steps, I felt
no pain—then the first block and then the first mile. I
couldn't believe I had completed a mile. One mile became
two, and as I was running back up to my house at the end
of my three-mile journey, I knew God was watching over me.
Ecstatic, I ran into my kitchen and shouted to my wife

that God had healed my foot, and tomorrow I would be able
to run the marathon. That was the first miracle of this
journey.

Tony

Think It Through

1. What physical problems have you encountered in running? How soon
   did you deal with them? What did you do?
2. What warning signs have you sensed recently in your relationship with
   God?
3. How will you respond to those signals? How will you deal with those
   issues?
4. What will be your first step?

On Running

Why is cross-training important?

The main value of cross-training is helping to reduce injury. By doing alternate activities, you can decrease the risk of overusing a muscle, take the
pressure off your knees, and increase your aerobic capacity as well. Biking
and swimming are good options for reducing the stress to knees and ankles.
Weight training will help to strengthen the muscles most used in running and
can increase speed and performance.

JOURNAL

_____

_____

_____

_____

_____

RUNNING LOG

	TIME	DISTANCE	WEATHER	NOTES
DAY 1				
DAY 2				
DAY 3				
DAY 4				
DAY 5				

DEAL WITH IT

Here's an interesting story about a marathon of sorts. Elijah had just seen God defeat the prophets of the false god Baal in a dramatic showdown on Mt. Carmel. Soon thereafter, he advised King Ahab to return to the capital city ahead of an impending storm. "Then the LORD gave special strength to Elijah. He tucked his cloak into his belt and ran ahead of Ahab's chariot all the way to the entrance of Jezreel" (1 Kings 18:46), a distance of about six miles.

But when word reached Queen Jezebel about what had happened to her prophets, she was furious and vowed to kill Elijah. So he ran again, this time for his life, all the way to Beersheba. Elijah was spent and needed physical and emotional healing:

Elijah was afraid and fled for his life. He went to Beersheba, a town in Judah, and he left his servant there. Then he went on alone into the wilderness, traveling all day. He sat down under a solitary broom tree and prayed that he might die. "I have had enough, LORD," he said. "Take my life, for I am no better than my ancestors who have already died."

Then he lay down and slept under the broom tree. But as he was sleeping, an angel touched him and told him, "Get up and eat!" He looked around and there beside his head was some bread baked on hot stones and a jar of water! So he ate and drank and lay down again.

Then the angel of the LORD came again and touched him and said, "Get up and eat some more, or the journey ahead will be too much for you."

So he got up and ate and drank, and the food gave him enough strength to travel forty days and forty nights to Mount Sinai, the mountain of God. There he came to a cave, where he spent the night. (1 KINGS 19:3-9)

At times our injuries may be emotional: burnout, sorrow, or as in the case of Elijah, depression. Just as with a physical issue, we need to heed the warning signs in this area and deal with the problem.

The Runner

In his service for God, Elijah had taken on the civil and religious authorities. And in the dramatic confrontation at Mt. Carmel, he had won. This was a tremendous victory for God and for Elijah. He must have been elated and also humbled at the demonstration of God's mighty power and the vindication of God's truth and his mission. During that time, he hadn't eaten or slept much; then he had run six miles, only to receive a death threat from Jezebel. So he ran again. Consider the physical and emotional toll. No wonder he was exhausted . . . and depressed. Elijah felt alone and abandoned, fearful and lost. What had happened to this courageous man of God?

Elijah was simply responding like a normal human being. We need rest; we need food; we need shelter; we need companionship—that's the way we're built, the way God made us. In Elijah's case, he had just come down from a spiritual high (an emotional valley often follows an emotional mountaintop), and he had powerful people trying to kill him, and all his running had exhausted him physically, making him even more vulnerable emotionally.

As is often the case, Elijah's physical and emotional needs were intertwined, and God dealt with both.

The Race

After Elijah stopped running, he asked God to take his life because he was depressed and lonely, and then he slept. Then he ate and drank what God had provided . . . and slept some more.

Eventually Elijah told God, "I have zealously served the LORD God Almighty. But the people of Israel have broken their covenant with you, torn down your altars, and killed every one of your prophets. I am the only one left, and now they are trying to kill me, too" (1 Kings 19:14). Did you hear that? Elijah felt totally isolated, alone. But God gave him new marching orders and assured him, "I will preserve 7,000 others in Israel who have never bowed down to Baal or kissed him!" (1 Kings 19:18)—that is, "You are not alone, and I am with you!"

We, too, can experience spiritual burnout, especially after pushing ourselves physically and achieving a victory. Often a crash follows. When that happens, we need to stop and recharge, which often means taking time to rest (even suspending our workouts or reducing our mileage) and eat. It also means spending time alone with God, honestly sharing our needs with him and allowing him to refresh our souls.

The Result

Physical, emotional, and spiritual burnout can come from an unrelenting schedule during which you skip meals and pull all-nighters or experience a series of relational crises, a crushing running/workout routine with no recovery time, a major life-change, or a combination of those factors. When you feel the crash coming, you need to deal with it—get off life's treadmill and get alone with God. Nourish yourself physically and spiritually. Rest . . . and come back stronger, ready to run!

My Story

Passionate runners often find that their running is closely tied to the very core of their being, their identity—"I'm a runner"; their view of personal success as an individual—"I was able to stick to my schedule this week!"; and even their sense of inner strength and well-being. All of these then come into question or are at least rattled by injury.

After running a half marathon a number of years ago, for which I had not properly prepared, I found my knees were so sore that I could hardly climb stairs or even walk up inclines. Later, while running a short sprint with some students I was coaching without warming up properly, I severely tore a hamstring. Mixed emotions accompanied both of these circumstances. On the one hand, a good running injury, especially something like sore knees from a half marathon, is almost a badge of honor. On the other hand, it shows that you are "weak" or maybe aging. Additionally, you are incapacitated for a period of time, and you are, for a period of time at least, not a "runner."

Throughout my life I have had to be careful not to let my running become too large a part of my identity. I must find my identity in Christ alone, not in performance, skill, or ability. This translates into many areas of my performance-based thinking, whether it be my vocation or my quest for spiritual growth or maturity. The "who I am" question must be answered before I slip into my running gear.

Rich

Think It Through

1. When has the combination of your responsibilities and workout schedule caused you to feel exhausted and burned-out physically? What did you do to recover?
2. When have other issues depleted your emotional reserves? How did you respond?
3. When have you experienced a spiritual high followed by a spiritual low? How did you get back on track?
4. What resources do you have to help you refresh and recharge your relationship with God?

On Running

What is proper rest and recovery?

Taking time for rest and recovery allows the muscles to take a break and heal. It also allows for replenishment of carbohydrates, our stored energy. Rest and recovery time differs for each person and each season. If you are training for an event, you probably will take more time for training than recovery. After the event, or during the off-season, you should be able to reduce your amount of training. Rest doesn't have to mean doing nothing. It can include cross-training, doing activities other than running. A basic plan for rest and recovery would be to take one day a week to completely rest and one day to cross-train. Experts recommend alternating hard and easy days as well.

JOURNAL

_____

_____

_____

_____

_____

RUNNING LOG

	TIME	DISTANCE	WEATHER	NOTES
DAY 1				
DAY 2				
DAY 3				
DAY 4				
DAY 5				

START SLOW

The principle of starting slow applies to workouts, but especially to long-distance races. Actually, unless you're a world-class runner, the first five miles in a marathon should be your slowest segment of the race. This pace allows the body to become acclimated to the run and keeps runners from using up their stored resources and burning out.

Centuries ago, King Solomon observed, "The fastest runner doesn't always win the race, and the strongest warrior doesn't always win the battle" (Ecclesiastes 9:11). His words often prove true, as some runners get caught up in the moment and run hard at the start only to pay for it later.

A bit later, Solomon made the parallel with the spiritual life. Addressing young people, he wrote, "Don't let the excitement of youth cause you to forget your Creator. Honor him in your youth before you grow old and say, 'Life is not pleasant anymore'" (Ecclesiastes 12:1).

The Living Bible paraphrases the last part of the verse this way: "before the evil years come—when you'll no longer enjoy living." To put that in running terms, "before you hit the wall, and you'll no longer enjoy running!"

The Runner

Cheri had put in her miles, rain or shine, and was ready for her first marathon. On race day, she did just as she had planned as to when she got up, what she ate, when she got to the staging area, and how she warmed up. Her friends and family were posted at critical points along the racecourse, ready to cheer her on. And she wore her watch and had her race plan around her wrist to make sure she was on track. She wanted to average nine-minute miles, a nice pace for her that she had been able to maintain in her long training runs. Cheri knew she should start slow and stick to ten-minute miles for the first five.

Bunched with her group at the start, Cheri saw a variety of runners, men and women, old, young, and in-between, of varying heights and weights, some wearing rather colorful outfits. She felt the competitive urge as she figured out who she should be able to beat. Everyone waited in nervous anticipation. Then the gun sounded, and they were off—thousands of feet pounding the pavement. As she swerved around slower runners, she found herself pushing ahead—and she felt great! But then she remembered, "Start slow!" and she was shocked to see that she had zipped through the first mile. Although she hated to do it, and sure didn't feel like it, Cheri slowed to her ten-minute-per-mile pace and suddenly became one of the slower runners being passed left and right.

Twenty miles later, however, she passed most of those runners and felt as if she still had enough to finish. And she did—for a personal best.

The Race

Excitement and expectations run high at the start of every race. Runners can easily get swept up in all the enthusiasm and with adrenaline pumping, tear off at the sound of the gun. Discipline is needed to maintain the correct, slower pace, even as others pass. Wise and experienced runners know the start is just the beginning, with many miles to follow. And if they want to finish well—or at all—they had better start slow, stretch when needed, and hydrate early (when they don't feel like it).

Life's marathon follows a similar route. When we're young, as Solomon reminds us, we can easily get caught up in the excitement, running this way and that, expending lots of energy with little thought for serious matters such as God or the future. But eventually "the evil years" of old age hit us when "life is not pleasant anymore." Nothing is sadder than listening to a bitter old person who looks back on life with regrets, voicing, "What if . . . ?" and "If only . . . !" Instead, we ought to honor our Creator right from the start so we can run our race with him. Then, nearing the finish, we can look back at a race well run with no regrets.

The Result

"Starting slow" in life means being serious about education, learning life skills, building solid relationships, and getting grounded in God's Word. We easily become impatient and try to hurry along the process, but these things take time. If you're young, the lesson is clear.

If you have blown past those years and are further down the road, you may still need to slow down, to stretch a bit and take nourishment. God wants to do his work in you, and he wants you to finish well.

My Story

Have you ever run in the early morning when the world is still asleep, when the sun has yet to rise and the darkness is lit by only a neighbor's porch light? You hear and see the things that the bright eyes of daylight don't reveal: the silence of a neighborhood still dreaming, the patter of your feet as you glide along a deserted street, the hoot of an owl greeting your day. The multitudes of stars fill the sky and sparkle as if freshly polished just for you. The mist rising above the neighborhood pond lends an eerie quality to the morning. And a mailbox is shadowed so it appears as a bystander cheering you on. Yes, running is a one-person sport, but I believe God is sharing himself each and every time we go out for one more run.

Mary

Think It Through

1. Why is a relatively slow start important in a long-distance race?
2. What factors influence young people to start too fast in life? When have you seen someone struggle in middle or late life because of that fast start?
3. When are you tempted to "forget your Creator"?
4. What does "starting slow" mean for you at this stage of life?

On Running

Why is water so important?

Water is vital to the body's cooling system. When you exercise, your internal body temperature increases and your body needs a way to cool off. One of the ways your body cools is through sweat. As you perspire, the sweat evaporates and allows you to stay cool. Without enough water, you can't sweat as much, so you can't cool your skin temperature. The increase in skin temperature causes your core temperature to increase as well. Taking in plenty of water before, during, and after exercise is very important—your body does not make water; it only conserves it.

JOURNAL

RUNNING LOG

	TIME	DISTANCE	WEATHER	NOTES
DAY 1				
DAY 2				
DAY 3				
DAY 4				
DAY 5				

START SLOW

Every race has rhythm, strategy, and execution. As we've been discussing, for most marathon runners their first five miles should be their slowest segment of the race. The stretch from mile six through fifteen should be the fastest, where the runner gets into a groove and hits his or her stride. From sixteen to twenty the runner should hold steady, and from twenty-one to twenty-six the runner should do the best he or she can, depending on the remaining physical and emotional reserves. Then comes the end of the race—with the goal in sight, the runner gives every ounce of strength to finish well. Each race has a time to run slow and a time to run fast.

Life has rhythms as well, and each life has a time to run slow and a time to run fast. Slowing down can be tough for many because we're geared to get going, move quickly, and work hard to accomplish our goals. But we aren't designed to go, go, go nonstop. We need hours and days at a much slower pace; we need rest. That's why God created the Sabbath, a day of rest. In the rhythm of life, we need to be still and be patient. David wrote, "Wait patiently for the LORD. Be brave and courageous. Yes, wait patiently for the LORD" (Psalm 27:14).

The Runner

Although he was born first, few years separate his siblings—all five of them. So his growing-up years were fun but a bit chaotic as Mom and Dad tried to shepherd the family. Every meal was an adventure, and eventually church and school activities and events packed the schedule.

As he matured, so did his electronics collection. At first he had just a radio, which he turned on as soon as he entered his bedroom. The family had one television set at first, but eventually they appeared in three or four rooms, with channels multiplying from the basic five or six to hundreds. The transistor radios of his childhood gave way to Walkmans, which gave way to MP3 players. And life moved on, faster every year. These days all the information he needs—and much of the entertainment—is at his fingertips with his phone, a constant companion. And now that he's immersed in a career, he has to be available at all times, receiving and sending calls, e-mails, and texts.

"Wait patiently" to hear from God—nearly impossible in this information-overloaded, noise-cluttered, and entertainment-saturated world.

The Race

Most believers would say they want to know God's will and ways—they want to hear from him. But we can't hear much of anything in all the noise of life. With schedules packed full of events and obligations, we race through every day honking, talking, texting, and tweeting. Even ministry events—services, meetings, socials, choirs, and classes—can hinder a relationship with God. At times we can be so busy doing, doing, doing that we neglect just "being." We're moving quickly through life but away from him without even realizing it. We need to slow down, take a breath, and listen. The Lord says, "Be still, and know that I am God! I will be honored by every nation. I will be honored throughout the world" (Psalm 46:10).

Just as at the beginning of a race when you have to think about your pace and consciously choose to start slow, finding time to "wait patiently" begins with a decision and needs to be intentional. This won't just happen—we won't suddenly encounter extended quiet, a significant gap in the schedule—because we are so easily caught up in each day's excitement and busyness. We need to choose to "be still."

The Result

Don't let the race of life set your pace for life. Build Sabbath into your schedule (regular times to slow down), be patient, be still, and listen to what God is saying. Walk away from the computer. Leave the iPod behind. Go to a place where you can almost feel the silence . . . and listen. Sometimes we can "be still" while running—if we're focused on God.

My Story

OCTOBER 17, 2007

Lord, my job is driving me crazy. I used to love it and felt called to it. I don't like who I am becoming, and the burden is too great. I have felt this way for eighteen months. Why am I so slow to trust you? Why am I so afraid of letting go? I'm staying home today. Let's go on a run together. . . .

Creation is screaming your name. The sun is breaking through the multicolored leaves you painted. The grass is damp with your breath. I'm sorry I ran for eighteen months. I can't run anymore—you take my breath away. I'm tired of running—I'm on my knees before you—on holy ground, face buried, tears flowing. I crawl to a huge stone next to the river. Your altar—I'm yours—I surrender all—my life is not my own—use me. You are my only treasure. I'm scared, Lord. No regrets!

(Copied from my journal, the day I transitioned from commodities trader to, eventually, youth pastor.)

Don P.

Think It Through

1. What noise fills your life? What activities, responsibilities, and events fill your schedule?
2. Why do you find slowing down so difficult?
3. When have you taken an extended period of time to listen to God speaking to you?
4. What can you do to carve out more personal time for God in your life?

On Running

How does my personality affect my performance?

Our personalities determine how we adjust to our environment, and each person responds differently and uniquely. Your psychological core is the most basic you—your feelings, self-concept, and so forth—the hardest area to get to know, but the most stable. Your personality traits will affect, therefore, how you typically respond to your environment. The more intense and competitive a person is, the more persistent that runner will be, obviously affecting his or her performance in a workout or race.

JOURNAL

_____

_____

_____

_____

_____

_____

_____

_____

RUNNING LOG

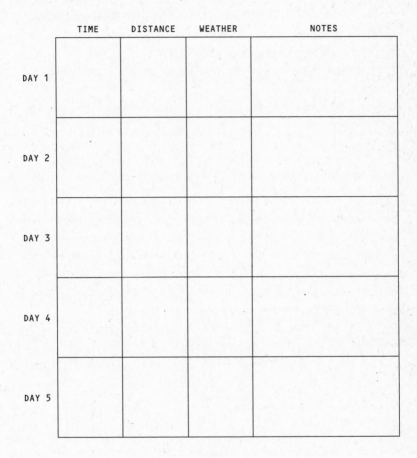

	TIME	DISTANCE	WEATHER	NOTES
DAY 1				
DAY 2				
DAY 3				
DAY 4				
DAY 5				

CHOOSE YOUR OWN PACE

Gather a group of runners and you'll discover many similarities in purposes, goals, motivations, nutrition, and favorite time of the day to run. But their differences are numerous and dramatic. Beyond the obvious ones of sex, age, and size, they also differ in running styles, routines, strides, and physical strengths and weaknesses—to name a few. We know that no two human beings are exactly alike, and the same can be said for runners. That's why each runner should establish running goals, a training schedule, and a racing pace that are appropriate for him or her. A six-foot-three-inch, 230-pound, forty-year-old business executive shouldn't expect to run like a 110-pound world-class runner from Kenya. That's obviously an extreme example, but the principle is the same. Each person should choose his or her own pace; copying someone else would be a mistake.

Individual believers vary as well, even though they may look similar, be in the same age group, come from the same socioeconomic and educational background, and go to the same church. Copying another person's spiritual race strategy would also be a mistake. Paul tells us:

*Don't copy the behavior and customs of this world, but let God
transform you into a new person by changing the way you think.
Then you will learn to know God's will for you, which is good
and pleasing and perfect.*

   *Because of the privilege and authority God has given me, I give
each of you this warning: Don't think you are better than you
really are. Be honest in your evaluation of yourselves, measuring
yourselves by the faith God has given us.* (ROMANS 12:2-3)

The Runner

"We'll run together," Jan told her friend Sue over coffee. They had
both decided to enter the big marathon coming up in six months in
the neighboring state. So they decided on a workout schedule and
held each other accountable to keep it. Seldom could they actually
train together because of their family and work situations. But they
had a goal and were working faithfully toward reaching it. And they
had compared their times for various runs—not the same, but close
enough, especially at the beginning. Eventually the gap in times wid-
ened, but they simply wrote off the slower time as running in the
afternoon instead of the morning or another reason or two.

   Race day arrived. They had driven to the city the night before and
stayed at a hotel near the starting line. They were ready to go on that
crisp and overcast morning. The gun sounded, and along with the
other five thousand or so runners, they took off, starting slow, as was
their plan. But at about the 10K mark, where they should have been
picking up the pace, Jan found herself struggling to keep up, and Sue
was frustrated as she kept looking back to find Jan, not wanting to lose
her in the sea of runners. At an aid station a couple of miles later, Jan
said through gulps of water, "You go on—run your pace. I'll see you
at the finish line."

   Reluctantly, Sue agreed, and they kept running. Both finished, Sue
about twenty minutes before Jan.

The Race

Although Jan and Sue had much in common and were highly moti-vated to run together, their differences put them on separate running paces. Yet both were successful—each one reached her goal. People are different.

According to our Romans 12 passage, we shouldn't "copy the behavior and customs of this world." We should be different on the inside, in worldview, perspective, values, and more; and those dif-ferences should affect how we look on the outside—our attitudes and actions. God is changing the way we think, how we approach life. So why would we even be tempted to copy the pace and style of worldly "runners"? But Paul also issues this warning: "Don't think you are better than you really are." Overrating ourselves will only get us into trouble. (That would be like the middle-aged business-man thinking he can run a sub-three-hour marathon.) Instead, we need to take a realistic and honest personal inventory, measuring ourselves by God's standards. If we're honest with ourselves, we know our strengths and weaknesses, our triumphs and tragedies, and our dreams and disasters.

In addition, each person has a unique blend of abilities, talents, and spiritual gifts (the focus of Romans 12:4-8). Instead of copying someone else and trying to use what we don't have, we should use the gifts we have for God's glory, setting our own spiritual pace.

We are also painfully aware of where we need help with our per-sonal set of problems and challenges. These vary greatly from person to person as well. The marriage challenges for a newlywed are quite different from someone who has just celebrated his or her fortieth anniversary. Parents of teenagers will have a whole new set of questions than when their kids were toddlers. Someone facing the severe illness or death of a loved one will need spiritual resources that others take for granted.

Choose your own pace.

The Result

Setting a personal pace in the Christian race will involve finding and using the appropriate resources, including wise counsel from other believers who have already traveled this stretch of the race. It will mean identifying and using *your* spiritual gifts:

> *Just as our bodies have many parts and each part has a special function, so it is with Christ's body. We are many parts of one body, and we all belong to each other.*
>
> *In his grace, God has given us different gifts for doing certain things well. So if God has given you the ability to prophesy, speak out with as much faith as God has given you. If your gift is serving others, serve them well. If you are a teacher, teach well. If your gift is to encourage others, be encouraging. If it is giving, give generously. If God has given you leadership ability, take the responsibility seriously. And if you have a gift for showing kindness to others, do it gladly.* (ROMANS 12:4-8)

Choose your own pace.

My Story

I'm a runner, but I'm not a marathoner. To call myself one, I would need to have run 26.2 miles in a race. To get to this point, a runner needs eighteen weeks of focused training. To be ready to train, many coaches advise three months of building a base—easy running to get into basic fitness. Yearly I tell my friends, "This year." And yearly I don't do it. I cannot decide on race day to run a marathon.

Am I a marathoner in matters of Christian service? Some ministries, like mowing a widow's lawn, can be jumped into headlong, like a 5K road race. Other ministries, like

translating the Bible into a new language, require years
of training and research. This year?

Anthony

Think It Through

1. When are you tempted to "copy the behaviors and customs of this
   world"?
2. Think of three or four runners you know. How do they differ in running
   ability, endurance, and motivation? Think of three or four of your
   Christian friends. How do they differ in spiritual giftedness?
3. As you set your spiritual pace, what resources do you need?
4. What can you do to better utilize your spiritual gifts in serving God and
   building up his church?

On Running

How does my perception of my ability affect my performance?

How you see yourself in terms of ability affects how you perform in many areas,
including running. A low perception of your ability will decrease your effort,
persistence, and performance. In other words, if you don't think you can run
very well or very far, you won't try as hard. On the other hand, a high perception
will increase your effort, persistence, and performance. After reaching certain
goals, however, those low perceptions can improve, along with performance.
A positive and realistic perception leads to a positive performance.

JOURNAL

_____

_____

_____

_____

_____

RUNNING LOG

	TIME	DISTANCE	WEATHER	NOTES
DAY 1				
DAY 2				
DAY 3				
DAY 4				
DAY 5				

CHOOSE YOUR OWN PACE

A runner's pace is personal, that is, it should be matched to his or her abilities, physical attributes, and goals. Runners shouldn't try to run exactly like anyone else. But that doesn't mean that a runner should never try to run faster. Actually, until the body begins to break down or wear down (through injury, use, or old age), experienced runners will tend to improve in speed and endurance. Putting in the miles with a regular running routine will increase endurance. And gradually pushing personal pace for certain distances will improve speed. Obviously this has limits—eventually every runner will reach the end of his or her resources. But serious runners want to improve. They love setting a new personal record for a race or a specific distance.

Wanting to improve is a commendable desire in every area of life. Jesus spoke to this desire when addressing the church at Thyatira. Before listing his complaints about the church and explaining what corrective action had to be taken, Jesus complimented them: "I know all the things you do. I have seen your love, your faith, your service, and your patient endurance. And I can see your constant improvement in all these things" (Revelation 2:19).

That almost sounds like a running coach: "You've been improving in every aspect of the sport, especially your endurance. That's good. Keep it up!"

God expects us to make strides in our relationship with him.

The Runner

Jon was a freshman phenom. With a willowy frame, his long legs ate up the yards, and his endurance was well beyond his fourteen years. Coach Taylor had spotted the boy at the first workout and soon moved him off the freshman cross-country squad to junior varsity. Coach was confident that he had a potential state champion on his team. Under his care, if this young man would work hard . . . well, the coach could dream, couldn't he?

Jon loved to run, and he especially loved to win races. And he was doing that—regularly—without much trouble. But Jon had other interests, most notably a girl he had met near the end of the fall season. She had come to his meets and had become one of his biggest fans. So while Coach had given Jon and the others an off-season training schedule, Jon hadn't paid much attention to it, with his attention diverted elsewhere.

The next fall, Jon's lack of training became obvious. Instead of showing improvement, his times were actually slower than the year before. So he and Coach Taylor had a little talk. Coach explained the potential he saw in Jon and that Jon would need to push himself to reach it. "Running comes easy for you, son," he said, "so you'll be tempted to slack off, to do only what you need to get by . . . and you'll probably still win your share of meets. But think of what you could accomplish if you *really tried*!" Coach went on to challenge Jon to keep working and keep improving, and Jon agreed to give it a shot, to do his best.

Two years later, he stood on the victory podium—he was state champion.

The Race

Jon's girlfriend wasn't the problem, just an excuse. Although Jon had all that potential, he was ignoring it and would have wasted it if Coach hadn't stepped in.

We expect to grow in every area of life as we get older and gain education and experience. Sometimes that happens naturally (as in physical growth, for example); but at times we have to work at it.

When the apostle Paul learned how the believers in Corinth were acting, he was not happy. They should have been much more spiritually mature than their actions indicated. So he wrote:

> *Dear brothers and sisters, when I was with you I couldn't talk to you as I would to spiritual people. I had to talk as though you belonged to this world or as though you were infants in the Christian life. I had to feed you with milk, not with solid food, because you weren't ready for anything stronger. And you still aren't ready, for you are still controlled by your sinful nature. You are jealous of one another and quarrel with each other. Doesn't that prove you are controlled by your sinful nature? Aren't you living like people of the world? When one of you says, "I am a follower of Paul," and another says, "I follow Apollos," aren't you acting just like people of the world?* (1 CORINTHIANS 3:1-4)

Did you catch that? Paul was saying, "Stop acting like babies and grow up!" The Corinthian believers had chosen their own pace, all right, but it was much slower than it should have been.

The Result

Sometimes looking back can give us perspective, looking back to what we were like then and seeing how far we've come. When you first gave your life to Christ, you had an outlook on life and goals for the future. Certainly those must have changed. You also may have had sinful habits that you needed to stop. And where were you in your Bible study and prayer life? Hopefully you've seen improvements and growth in all those areas. If not, you may need to become more serious about your spiritual workouts.

My Story

After running the Chicago Marathon for the first time and having to wait forty-five minutes in line for the Porta-Potty, I decided that if I did it again, I would be a charity runner so that I could have access to Charity Village, where each charity has its own private Porta-Potties—with no lines! Clearly this is a pretty lame reason for becoming a charity runner, but doing so has changed my running perspective immensely. The past four years I have run Chicago for the American Cancer Society, and each year I have even more motivation for my training, the race, and my fund-raising. Everyone knows someone who has been affected by cancer. Sadly I have had two very dear friends die of the disease just this past year, not to mention the handful of friends I have who are currently battling cancer in some form or another.

This past year was especially tough to train. I thought the heat would never let up—I do not run well in the heat. In fact, I would much prefer to run in twenty degrees and snow or forty degrees and rain than to run in anything over seventy degrees. My body just slows down, my legs become like lead, I feel nauseous, my head hurts, and I can't imagine running any distance longer than three miles. But run long I must, as my training calls for fourteen-, sixteen-, eighteen-, and twenty-mile runs, despite the hot, humid weather. Because my body did not want to cooperate, I had to dig deep and rely on my mind and prayer to get me through these runs and through this year's Chicago Marathon, which had temperatures close to ninety degrees!

During those particularly hot runs, I thought about and

prayed for the family and friends who have had to deal with
so much more. Thinking about their pain—pain far greater
than my temporary discomfort; the chemotherapy that made
them sick for days on end, far more so than my bout of
nausea for a few miles; the daily battles they have faced,
many of which never went away—I have been humbled and
honored to run in their honor and memory. So whenever it got
a little tough for me and I wanted to quit, I told myself to
put on my big-girl pants and get going.

I try to remember these things during the struggles of
day-to-day life, as well. When I think of what Christ has
done for me, what he endured on the cross so that I could
have everlasting life, I find it hard to complain and easy
to be filled with gratitude. Whether dealing with a blister
at mile twenty-five, a coworker with a bad attitude, or the
daily balancing act of work, family, laundry, cleaning,
cooking, and volunteering, I count my blessings and am
grateful that I can handle it. I thank God that he gave me
the ability, desire, and enjoyment of running!

Ellen

Think It Through

1. In what ways has your running improved since you began?
2. How have you grown and matured in your Christian life?
3. In what faith areas have you been coasting, taking it easy? Why?
4. What can you do to improve your "love, faith, service, and patient
   endurance"?

On Running

What causes stress and anxiety in competition?

Anxiety is an emotional response to stresses that can consist of combina-
tions of feelings, cognitions, and physiological changes. A number of factors
can cause stress and anxiety in a sporting situation. A person may be afraid
of defeat, lack confidence in his or her ability, or have a form of stage

fright (fear of performing in front of others). Anxiety may be heightened by the intensity of the competition, the importance of the event (and consequences of defeat), and the fear of the unknown. A certain level of anxiety is normal and may even help the athlete do better. But great anxiety can be detrimental, almost paralyzing.

JOURNAL

_____

_____

_____

_____

_____

RUNNING LOG

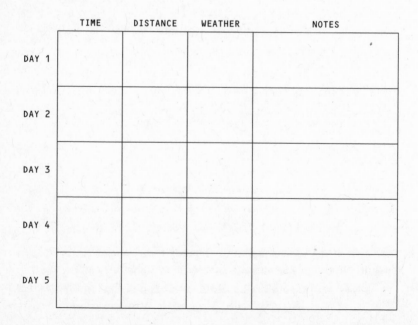

	TIME	DISTANCE	WEATHER	NOTES
DAY 1				
DAY 2				
DAY 3				
DAY 4				
DAY 5				

RUN THE ROUTE

Race organizers lay out a route of the appropriate distance, from start to finish. But they consider much more than just the required distance. In designing the route, they look at the race from a number of perspectives: the community (how it will affect traffic, businesses, and so forth); the spectators (their ability to see runners and get from one point to another along the course); race necessities (the availability of parking at the start and finish, placement of aid stations, shuttles between start and finish, huge crowds at the start and finish, room for first-aid tents, sponsors' booths at the finish); and of course, the runners (fair course—wide enough with no potholes, interesting sites, some challenges).

The goal for any runner should be to run the entire course in the desired time. Certainly, runners would like to win or place high, if not in the entire race, at least in their age group. But most are pleased when they set a personal record (PR). Whether the race is a 5K or a marathon, runners learn much about themselves as they draw on their emotional, mental, and physical reserves; push themselves to the limit; and persevere.

As we run life's race, we have the same experience, especially when we have to draw on our spiritual reserves. We discover truths about ourselves and God as we learn to rely on him and his strength. That was Paul's prayer for his Christian brothers and sisters in Ephesus (we also looked at a portion of this passage in Week 1):

> *When I think of all this, I fall to my knees and pray to the Father, the Creator of everything in heaven and on earth. I pray that from his glorious, unlimited resources he will empower you with inner strength through his Spirit. Then Christ will make his home in your hearts as you trust in him. Your roots will grow down into God's love and keep you strong. And may you have the power to understand, as all God's people should, how wide, how long, how high, and how deep his love is. May you experience the love of Christ, though it is too great to understand fully. Then you will be made complete with all the fullness of life and power that comes from God.* (EPHESIANS 3:14-19)

We begin to understand God's love and power as we run the route he has marked out for us.

The Runner

Have you heard the story about Rosie Ruiz? On April 21, 1980, she seemed to have recorded the fastest time ever for a woman in the Boston Marathon when she crossed the finish line at 2:31:56. Race officials were suspicious, however, because she didn't seem very tired after such a grueling race. More important, no one could recall seeing Rosie during the race, and she certainly would have stood out if she had been one of the leading women runners. But several spotters at various checkpoints didn't remember seeing her in the first group of women. She also didn't appear in any pictures or video footage.

Then two Harvard students said they remembered seeing Ruiz jump out of a crowd of spectators, half a mile from the finish. So she hadn't run the entire course—just the last half mile.

A bit later, a woman said she had met Ruiz on the subway during the New York City Marathon and had walked with her from the subway to the race. She had lost touch with Ruiz after that but came forward when she heard of Ruiz's dubious Boston win. According to this woman, they had walked to the finishing area, where Ruiz had said she was an injured runner. Her time for the New York City Marathon had qualified her for Boston.

Today, Rosie Ruiz is remembered as a cheater. She took a shortcut to the finish (in both races) and was disqualified and disgraced.

The Race

Rosie wasn't concerned about actually persevering and completing a marathon, about achieving an earned PR, or about learning life lessons. Her goal was to win and to be recognized for a fast time in the race. So she took a shortcut; she cheated and was disqualified.

Shortcuts are tempting. Some take them in classes, cheating on tests. Some do this in manufacturing and sell inferior products. Some even take this approach in relationships. Though they may seem to win at first, eventually they are disqualified; they lose.

Paul took this truth about shortcuts seriously. We looked at this passage in Week 4, but listen again to what he says about being disciplined in life: "I discipline my body like an athlete, training it to do what it should. Otherwise, I fear that after preaching to others I myself might be disqualified" (1 Corinthians 9:27). Paul didn't want to be a hypocrite, urging others to live one way while he didn't live that way himself. No shortcuts for Paul . . . and no disqualification. He ran the route God had set before him.

The Result

Unfortunately, some people who claim to follow Christ just want to be known as being "spiritual." They talk a good game and make public their devotional life, service projects, and financial donations, but their lifestyle is phony, superficial. They have substituted devotion to self and personal glory for devotion to Christ.

The spiritual life has no shortcuts. But that's what's so great about it. As we run God's route for us, around corners, avoiding obstacles, over hills, in valleys, and in difficult conditions, we grow deeper and stronger and learn to depend on him.

My Story

My sister and I knew the day would be wet before it even began. We were running our third half marathon together, my second time on this course. The rain poured as we waited in traffic to get into the parking lot. While we were stopped, we put on our shoes and numbers because it was getting dangerously close to race time. We finally pulled into the lot ten minutes after the start and hustled out of the car.

To warm up, we jogged to the start line. As we crossed an empty parking lot, wondering why we couldn't have parked there, we ended up in almost knee-deep water, thankful that our timing chips were on our numbers and not on our shoes. It didn't feel like a race at all as we crossed the start line with no one else even in sight.

Because we were running into the wind and rain was pelting our faces, we spent most of the first few miles looking at the road just in front of our feet. We started to catch up to some runners near the end of the second mile. We turned one corner and were hit with such a blast of wind that it felt as if we had to lean forty-five degrees to keep from blowing over. Each time I picked up my right foot, the wind blew it into my left leg.

Before mile seven, we started to see runners coming back along the course. We were confused because we knew that wasn't how the course was laid out. Then they turned us toward the finish line, explaining that the course

had been changed. More and more runners were coming by.
Finally one announced that the course had been closed and
that everyone, even the full marathon runners, had to stop
at ten miles.

As we finished, we felt cheated, having run only ten
miles after not even getting to start with everyone.
Heavy rains had fallen the whole time and showed no
signs of stopping. To say that we were wet would be an
understatement. Not a millimeter of us was dry.

We got our medals and headed for the bus line to get
our ride back to the starting point and our car. I was
glad to be warm and out of the rain and wind . . . or so
I thought. Every time the bus turned right, I got poured
on through the emergency exit in the roof! Well, that
had to be as wet as I could get, right?

Not so fast! As we walked back to our vehicle, a
passing car drove through a puddle and drenched us from
the waist down. We found ourselves looking heavenward and
asking, "Really? We weren't wet enough yet?"

When we got back to my sister's house, still feeling
cheated that we had done all the training and hadn't been
able to run the whole race, we were met by her husband,
who ushered us over to the computer to see pictures of
all the flooding that was happening because of the storm.
In the end I got to spend an extra day with my sister
because the trains were canceled due to the tracks being
underwater in places.

God did not keep us from getting wet, but he sure
protected us throughout the storm! And he gave me a
strange running adventure that I'll never forget.

Katy

Think It Through

1. When have you seen someone cheat in an athletic contest? What do
   you think motivated him or her? What happened?

2. What kind of shortcuts are believers tempted to make in the Christian life? What makes them so appealing?
3. When has God's route for your life seemed tough? What did you learn about yourself and about God by staying the course and running through those difficult times?
4. What can you do to make sure that you run the route God has laid out for you?

On Running

How can I reduce my anxiety?

First of all, you need to increase your personal awareness. What causes you to have anxiety? Which circumstances? How about the way you feel about yourself? Next, realize how these things intertwine. Become aware of your physical response to anxiety; for example, do you get butterflies before you compete? Develop a relaxation technique, and have someone help you grow your confidence. Finally, realize that fear is natural; you need to face your fears, or they will paralyze you.

JOURNAL

_____

_____

_____

_____

_____

_____

_____

_____

RUNNING LOG

	TIME	DISTANCE	WEATHER	NOTES
DAY 1				
DAY 2				
DAY 3				
DAY 4				
DAY 5				

RUN THE ROUTE

Wise athletes, runners included, listen to their coaches and do what they say, trusting the coaches' wisdom. That's what God told Joshua as he was taking over as leader of the Israelites on their march to the Promised Land. Moses had been the leader and had left instructions for Joshua. So God told him:

> *Be strong and courageous, for you are the one who will*
> *lead these people to possess all the land I swore to their*
> *ancestors I would give them. Be strong and very courageous.*
> *Be careful to obey all the instructions Moses gave you. Do*
> *not deviate from them, turning either to the right or to*
> *the left. Then you will be successful in everything you do.*
> (JOSHUA 1:6-7)

Twice in this passage, God encouraged Joshua to be strong and courageous. That makes sense because Joshua had been given a tough assignment. Then God told Joshua to follow his "coach" Moses' instructions, emphasizing that point with this statement: "Do not deviate from them, turning either to the right or to the left." That sounds like a runner, keeping focused on the course and the goal.

Along the racecourse, especially over long distances, runners will encounter many distractions—thoughts, obstacles, spectators, sounds, and sights. Any of these can slow a runner down and may even get him or her off course. Successful runners stay focused as they run the route.

The Runner

This was the day for Trevor's longest run yet—five miles. Until now he had been a regular jogger and had hit the three-mile mark a couple of times. But he decided to make the move to the next level, and he knew he was ready. He was excited about the challenge, but was dreading it as well, figuring he'd probably be exhausted at the end.

So Trevor put on his running outfit and laced up his shoes in the garage. On his way out the door, he spotted a rake on the lawn that he had forgotten to put away after raking the leaves the previous afternoon. Walking to the rake, he saw some papers and a plastic bottle that had blown into his yard during the night, so he grabbed the trash and the rake and started back to the garage. The plastic bottle reminded him that he probably should grab his water bottle and bring it out for after his run, so he went in to get it.

Then he thought, *I probably should eat an energy bar because I'll be running longer today*, and he went to the pantry to retrieve one. As he walked back to the door, Trevor noticed he had tracked in some leaves and dirt from the yard. *Sally will kill me*, he thought. *I'd better take care of that right now before she gets home.* He removed his dirty shoes, got out the vacuum cleaner, and took care of the mess.

But thinking of his wife and her possible reaction reminded him that she had asked him to take the meat out of the freezer to thaw. *Phew—almost forgot*, he thought, as he quickly returned to the kitchen and put the meat on the counter.

He had just taken a few steps away when he decided he should probably put a paper towel under the package in case anything leaked out—but the holder was empty. *Where does she keep those towels?* Trevor wondered as he searched the kitchen.

Just then the phone rang. Trevor answered and took a lengthy message for his teenage daughter. "Now, where was I?" he muttered and resumed his search for the towels. . . .

The Race

At times you may have felt like Trevor—wanting to accomplish a goal, perhaps a long run, but dreading it at the same time. In the process, you become easily distracted. Hmmm—we can wonder if Trevor ever got started.

We've already looked at the issue of shortcuts—that's one tactic Satan uses to get us off our course of following Christ. But other distractions can cause problems. Sometimes something good can keep us from what is best for us, or a worthy pursuit can pull us away from the direction God wants us to go. That would be like a runner stopping to pose for pictures, to text a friend, to make a deposit at an ATM, or to have a political debate with a spectator in the middle of a race. Those aren't bad activities, but they would distract and impede the runner and keep him or her from reaching the goal. We may forgo worship for another activity, scrimp and save for a family vacation but stop tithing in the process, or even ignore someone in obvious need while rushing to choir practice. In other words, our priorities can get out of whack.

Other distractions can turn out to be detours and take us way off course.

The Result

Put yourself in Joshua's place and hear God's clear instructions: "Be strong and very courageous. Be careful to obey all the instructions [that I have given you]. Do not deviate from them, turning either to the right or to the left. Then you will be successful in everything you do."

God has given us his Word filled with timeless truths. Through it he tells us how to live, how to be successful for him—how to win his race. Don't be distracted. Run your route.

My Story

My friend Sam was big on running, and I would think, *Man, is he crazy!* Running had never been my thing. Personally, I thought it was suicide. But when the words "You should do cross-country" slipped from his mouth one day, I couldn't help but consider it.

I knew I needed more exercise. *Besides,* I told myself, *it will help me to have more energy for basketball and be the fastest one down the court.* Eventually I listened to that small voice in my head and decided that I *would* do cross-country in the fall.

When I started training in July, I could barely run a mile at my very slow jogging pace. But God wouldn't let me quit. I was completely motivated to keep at it, and I slowly improved. By the end of the summer I was able to run three miles, but I had no idea how slow my pace really was.

Cross-country began in late August. The exercise was basic, and I rolled my eyes at the many people I watched walk. But this confidence didn't last long. As my first full week of practice progressed, my legs began giving way, and my shins felt as if they had been glued to a hot stove. I developed shin splints in both of my legs, slowing me down and causing me to miss the first two meets of the season.

Frustrated, I wasn't giving up. I watched with my jaw locked as my best friend, Erin, who was also a beginner, rapidly progressed. She quickly became one of the best runners on our eighth-grade girls team. I was still stuck near the back.

After one meet where I came in third to last, I got

off the bus on the verge of tears. I couldn't take it. Why wasn't I improving as fast as everyone else? My shins were still throbbing, and I couldn't run on the weekends because I needed to give them a rest. I felt useless. But every time I thought about quitting, something stopped me. Imagining Erin's and Sam's disappointed faces kept me going. No matter what I did, I wasn't going to be a quitter.

At our last home meet, something changed. Instead of being frustrated with how badly I'd performed, I decided just to be happy with how hard I had worked. On the final stretch, my friend Kelly cheered me on alongside me, giving me the last bit of motivation I needed to finish in a full-out sprint. I wasn't letting the girl behind me beat me. I smiled as I finished. I had done it! I had left her completely in the dust. As I limped back to my team, I couldn't help but reflect on the way I had reacted when I'd finished.

The season soon came to an end. The weather during the conference meet was cold and windy. My legs felt frozen, wearing only running shorts. Halfway through the race, I developed horrible cramps in my calves that wouldn't go away. This was the most painful race yet.

But it was my best race of the season. I sprinted the final stretch, almost beating the girl far in front of me. Afterward, I had to put my arms behind my head to keep myself from throwing up. It was the fastest I had ever run two miles, and boy, was it satisfying!

Cross-country is probably the most frustrating, difficult sport I've ever done. In a way, I've grown to love it. God had his reasons for pushing me through this season—he always does. I've honestly enjoyed my running experience so far and know I'll always be running—maybe not on a cross-country team, but I'll always run. I'll never think of running as being a "suicidal" sport ever again.

Kaitlyn

Think It Through

1. What distractions have you encountered in races you've run?
2. When have you seen believers pulled off their spiritual course by giving in to temptations? When have you been tempted that way?
3. Which "good" activities have caused you to be distracted from pursuing the "best"?
4. What can you do to stay focused on doing what God wants, not "turning either to the right or to the left"?

On Running

What dietary goals should I have?

If you are running to lose weight, feel well, and do your best in races, dietary goals are important. As a consistent runner, you will need to consume food and calories differently than other people—different types and ratios. Your dietary goals should not just relate to your daily consumption, but also to how you eat prior to, during, and after a race. By having these goals (a plan), you'll likely feel better and see more success in your races and weight loss.

JOURNAL

_____

_____

_____

_____

_____

_____

_____

RUNNING LOG

	TIME	DISTANCE	WEATHER	NOTES
DAY 1				
DAY 2				
DAY 3				
DAY 4				
DAY 5				

MONITOR YOURSELF

We know our own bodies better than anyone else, except perhaps a doctor who has prodded, probed, and tested us. Unless we have an obvious external injury, we feel most of our pains *inside*; only we are aware of them. We also know which feelings to ignore, such as stiffness from sitting in a car on a long drive, the burning sensation after ingesting a hot pepper, the pain of scraping our knuckles against a brick wall, and other minor aches and irritations. But some sensations are like warning lights and should be taken seriously—a sudden severe headache, chest pains, blurred vision, and others. We monitor our physical well-being by being aware of what our bodies are telling us.

Self-monitoring is vital in working out (we discussed this in Week 17) and in running, especially during long-distance races. We need to be aware of the warning signals and take appropriate action— stopping to stretch, applying Vaseline, removing a layer of clothing, taking fluids, and so forth. We should also monitor how we're doing as we compare pace, time, and distance with our plan. Some runners wear heart monitors, and those with special needs have other medical devices.

Of course, these signals and monitors simply give us information. We still need to respond. Not only will this help us avoid injury, it will also make us better runners.

Self-monitoring is important in our spiritual lives as well. But here's a bulletin: God has given us an internal monitor—the Holy Spirit. Listen to this powerful truth:

> *You are not controlled by your sinful nature. You are controlled by the Spirit if you have the Spirit of God living in you. (And remember that those who do not have the Spirit of Christ living in them do not belong to him at all.)* (ROMANS 8:9)

Jesus said that the Holy Spirit will "convict the world of its sin, and of God's righteousness, and of the coming judgment" (John 16:8). Simply put, this means that the Holy Spirit will make us sensitive to sin and its consequences. He'll let us know when we're running off course and need to take corrective action—like a spiritual GPS.

The Runner

A. Hare was a natural athlete who could run circles around just about anyone. Running was so natural to him that he always seemed to be in motion. One day A. signed up for the local marathon. He knew he could do it . . . and he certainly was in shape. At the start, A. took off and was easily in the first pack of runners. He blew past the aid stations while others were slowing to grab some water. After a few miles A. felt a hot spot on one foot, but he thought, *That's nothing*, and kept running. A mile later his left hamstring felt a little tight, but he shrugged it off and kept running. In another couple of miles, both situations had worsened, and A. had to slow and sort of hop along.

T. Ortice also liked to run, but he wasn't very fast—just steady. T. had been looking forward to the marathon and had trained for three months; he knew he was ready. At the start, everyone seemed to get the jump on him, but he left and ran his usual slow but steady pace. Down the road a bit, T. felt a hot spot on one foot, so he stopped at an aid station and applied some petroleum jelly. He also was careful to drink fluids early because he knew he'd need the hydration later. When his hamstring felt a little tight, he stopped and stretched it out, not wanting to risk pulling it. And he kept running—not very fast, but steady.

Guess who finished the race?

The Race

Like T. Ortice, if we want to run well and finish the race, we need to monitor ourselves and heed the warning signals, especially what the Holy Spirit is telling us.

The Spirit will speak to us through our conscience, our internal moral compass, but he will also use godly preachers, teachers, writers, and leaders. God may whisper a warning through a Christian friend or shout one through a challenge or conflict. But most often, he speaks through his Word, which we've already discussed in Week 8.

"All Scripture is inspired by God and is useful to teach us what is true and to make us realize what is wrong in our lives. It corrects us when we are wrong and teaches us to do what is right" (2 Timothy 3:16), and "we must listen very carefully to the truth we have heard, or we may drift away from it" (Hebrews 2:1).

As we read Scripture, we learn about God and how he wants us to live. And in measuring our lives by his standards, we monitor ourselves.

The Result

This monitoring process isn't all negative. Certainly the Holy Spirit will convict us of sin and tell us to stop acting and thinking in the wrong ways. But he will also point us toward positive actions to take. God may urge us to help a person in need, share the gospel with a friend or coworker, donate generously to his work, or come alongside someone who's hurting.

Being sensitive to the Holy Spirit's urgings and hearing God's voice will keep us moving in the right direction and running well.

My Story

My first marathon was the Chicago Marathon, which had about thirty-eight thousand runners. I was in awe of the entire event. The shot went off, but it took me ten minutes just to get to the starting line. I was not sure how far I could run, but I knew that if I could make twenty miles, I could make it to the end.

I ran the first five miles on adrenaline, and it was awesome. The next five miles got a little tougher, and after about ten miles I knew I would need help to make it.

I had my cell phone with me and called one of my best friends, Phil. He knew I was training for the marathon but thought I wouldn't be able to run due to my foot injury. I let him know that I needed him to help me finish and asked if he could meet me at mile marker thirteen to run the rest of the way with me. Phil was in his car, about fourteen miles from the race. I knew it would be a long shot for him to make it there in time, but to my surprise he was waiting for me in front of St. Patrick's Church, just as we planned, to help me finish this journey. Phil is a good athlete but had not run more than a few miles at one time. But he ran the last thirteen miles with me, seemingly carrying me to the finish line.

Every time I hear the story of the four men who carried their sick friend to see Jesus, cutting a hole in the roof of the house and lowering him down, I think of my buddy Phil. I believe that because of his faith in God and in me, he was able to carry me through.

I learned a lot in this journey: how faith in God will

sustain us through thick and thin, how God wants us to put
our burdens and trust in him, and how we can be supported
by our friends and family.

Tony

Think It Through

1. When you run, to what warning signals are you sensitive? What changes
   have you made because of these signals and monitoring devices?
2. How has God used others to keep you on track?
3. What Bible passages has the Holy Spirit used recently to convict you of
   something you should or shouldn't do?
4. What can you do to better monitor yourself spiritually?

On Running

How do I lose water?

Runners lose water in a few ways. The most obvious is through sweat.
Sweating helps cool the body through evaporation. Water is also lost in
urine. As your sweat increases, your amount of urine will decrease. You can
also lose respiratory water, that is, through breathing. All this water loss
highlights the importance of hydration, especially during long runs and in
warm weather.

JOURNAL

RUNNING LOG

	TIME	DISTANCE	WEATHER	NOTES
DAY 1				
DAY 2				
DAY 3				
DAY 4				
DAY 5				

MONITOR YOURSELF

At times the monitoring process is proactive rather than reactive. That is, instead of waiting for an irritation to develop or a symptom to appear, we test ourselves to see how we're doing. It's much like the annual physical exam where the physician checks pulse, blood pressure, and so forth and orders blood and urine tests. We want to know ourselves better and discover any potential problems.

In running, increasing self-awareness might involve trying a new running routine—pushing ourselves to see how our legs, lungs, and heart will respond. It could include trying new gear to help weather the weather. It may mean asking a coach, personal trainer, or running buddy to analyze our running style and make suggestions for improvements. At times we need to take the initiative to learn more about ourselves.

Often the Bible tells us to test or examine ourselves, to be spiritually proactive. Addressing the exiled people of Judah, Jeremiah wrote:

Who can command things to happen without the Lord's permission? Does not the Most High send both calamity and good? Then why should we, mere humans, complain when we

are punished for our sins? Instead, let us test and examine our
ways. Let us turn back to the LORD. (LAMENTATIONS 3:37-40)

Centuries later, the apostle Paul challenged the believers in Corinth: "Examine yourselves to see if your faith is genuine. Test yourselves. Surely you know that Jesus Christ is among you; if not, you have failed the test of genuine faith" (2 Corinthians 13:5).

The Runner

Joanie sat in church, slumped in her seat until everyone stood for the songs, which she sang halfheartedly. This had not been a good morning. First, she had slept poorly and had greeted the day with a headache. Next, as she was getting dressed, she couldn't find the sweater she wanted to wear, so she had to change outfits. Then she had spilled milk on her dress at breakfast, causing her to change again. And to top it off, the road seemed to be filled with idiot drivers, and she pulled into the parking lot later than usual and had trouble finding a parking space. But at least she was in church. *That ought to count for something*, she thought.

During the sermon on Philippians 4:10-13, the pastor made a statement that got Joanie's attention: "Lack of contentment should be a warning light. If you're frustrated, irritated, joyless, and upset most of the time, something's wrong."

That's me! Joanie thought. *Paul suffered incredible hardships—shipwreck, numerous beatings, imprisonment, and more—yet he was content in Christ. And here I am upset and feeling sorry for myself over a few insignificant irritations.*

The Holy Spirit was speaking to Joanie through God's Word and her pastor . . . and she was paying attention.

The Race

A natural response to this idea of proactive spiritual testing would be "How? What are the warning lights?" Good questions!

We've seen that the Holy Spirit provides our internal monitoring system through his convicting work. And we've also seen that he speaks to us through Scripture. Putting those two truths together, we find perhaps the best location for spiritual indicators in Galatians 5:22-23. Here Paul describes the positive results, the "fruit" of the Spirit's work in our lives: "But the Holy Spirit produces this kind of fruit in our lives: love, joy, peace, patience, kindness, goodness, faithfulness, gentleness, and self-control."

If the Holy Spirit is supposed to be producing these qualities in us, then the *lack* of any of these should be an indicator that something isn't right.

The Result

Think these through, one at a time, asking the appropriate questions:

- Love—Do I respond to people, even those who irritate me, with love?
- Joy—Do I still feel the joy of my salvation (Psalm 51:8, 12), or have I become gloomy or fearful?
- Peace—Do I sense God's calm in my personal storms?
- Patience—Can I wait, or do I have to have everything *now*?
- Kindness—Do I treat others with understanding and respect?
- Goodness—Am I trying to do what's right, even if it costs me?
- Faithfulness—Do I keep my promises? Can people count on me?
- Gentleness—Am I approachable, or do people keep their distance because of my negative, intimidating attitude?
- Self-control—Am I able to keep my emotions in check and not swing to extremes in behavior?

If any of those warning lights are blinking, you should go immediately to your Manufacturer: Admit your problem and ask him to correct you on the inside, giving you new ability and strength to run his race.

My Story

As one who prefers endurance events, I end up enjoying many long workouts in preparation for race day. After most training days, I feel a terrific sense of accomplishment and well-being. On long training days, however, I sometimes find my efforts out of sync with my training needs. I push too hard, lose sight of my goals, and take the day beyond appropriate limits. I find myself overdoing it despite receiving a lot of well-intended advice from training partners, like "build your base" and "pace your training effort."

So lately, rather than allowing my efforts to rise during long runs or rides, I have taken a different approach: structure, discipline, and distraction. No more random workouts. A good strategy is to have a plan and try new approaches to hydration and nutrition during training. This deliberate switch helps me take the focus off speed and puts me in a much better place after the workout is over. So I experiment with different ways to fuel up, stay hydrated, and take in nutrition. Trying new ideas during training allows me to steer clear of hammering out the miles too fast and regretting it later.

This training approach came in handy during my half-ironman experience in Muncie, Indiana. I felt great on the swim despite the stormy water and made a quick transition to the bike. It rained 95 percent of the bike course, which made me feel deceivingly hydrated and cool. My core body temperature was good, but the trouble was staying adequately hydrated on the bike in preparation for the run. Starting any long run on a hydration deficit is a big mistake. I was able to force myself to consume a slurry of liquid nutrition and fluid electrolytes, which I had

learned to do on long training days. During the run, the
rain cleared, and the sun's hot rays pounded me. Learning
to consume fluids during training paid off during the
run, allowing me to finish healthy. Thank goodness, too,
for having training partners who hold me accountable and
consistent.

And as I have been told, sometimes less really is more.
So on long training days, I back off the speed, save
it for another day, remain confident in a more moderate
training effort, and try new approaches to endurance
essentials like hydration and calories.

What I have come to learn is that it is far more about
the journey than the actual event, anyway.

Don R.

Think It Through

1. When has a physical check-up alerted you to a problem or potential
   issue? What did you have to change (medication, diet, running routine,
   other)?
2. What other proactive steps have you taken to monitor yourself?
3. As you went through the "spiritual indicators" listed earlier, which
   warning lights were blinking?
4. What corrective action will you take?

On Running

Why do I have to drink water before and during workouts and races?

A big problem for runners is that often their water intake tends to be a lot
less than their water loss. Our bodies don't produce water; we only conserve
water. The amount of water used by an athlete depends on the sport, duration, and environmental conditions (for example, if you sweat a lot, you'll
need more water). All athletes need to rehydrate, even swimmers! So, if you
are doing a swim workout, remember to drink plenty of water because the
warmer the water, the more you sweat.

JOURNAL

_____

_____

_____

_____

_____

RUNNING LOG

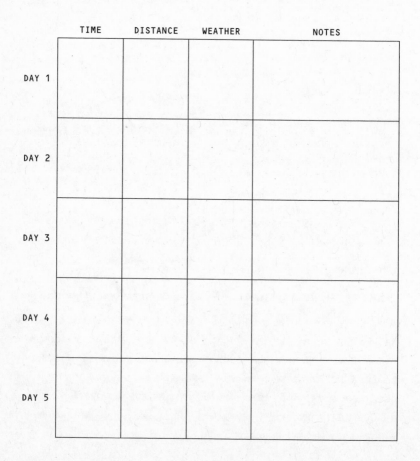

	TIME	DISTANCE	WEATHER	NOTES
DAY 1				
DAY 2				
DAY 3				
DAY 4				
DAY 5				

INCREASE YOUR SPEED

People run for a variety of reasons, and they vary greatly in body shapes and running styles. They may begin running by jogging a few blocks. Then, as they gain stamina and confidence, they lengthen those daily runs and increase their pace. Regardless of how long they go or how often, all runners recognize the difference between a run in the neighborhood and a race. By definition, a race implies competition with other runners and especially against the clock. Certainly many runners race to win, but most simply want to improve, to set a personal record. Some may, in fact, enter a race just for fun and for a T-shirt—that's fine. Usually, however, runners want to run strong and finish well. Besides the obvious physical preparation, this will mean running a smart race, which means knowing when to run faster.

We've already discussed warming up (stretching and getting ready to run) and running at the pace that is right for us. This involves starting slow (allowing the body to adjust to the run). But the next portion of the race should be where we pick up the pace. In a marathon, this would be miles six through fifteen. This doesn't mean sprinting—we still have a long way to go—but significantly bumping up our speed. We want to get into a groove and move along. We want to do our best.

The Bible has an interesting verse tucked into Ephesians. Speaking to servants, Paul writes, "Work with enthusiasm, as though you were working for the Lord rather than for people" (Ephesians 6:7).

Usually this verse is applied to how Christians perform their jobs, their secular employment. Instead of simply working to make a paycheck or to please an employer, we should work as if God is our boss.

He is.

And notice the first part of the verse: "Work with enthusiasm." This means working hard and doing our best. Paul is saying, in effect, "You have an audience of one." James seems to echo that thought when he talks about asking God for wisdom: "When you ask him, be sure that your faith is in God alone. Do not waver, for a person with divided loyalty is as unsettled as a wave of the sea that is blown and tossed by the wind" (James 1:6).

No divided loyalties—live (and run) for God alone.

The Runner

Jim Elliot had several hobbies as a boy and loved sledding down the mountain near his home (an extreme sport of that day). In high school, he played football and participated in many other activities. After high school, Jim enrolled at Wheaton College in Illinois, where he competed on the wrestling team. Jim was known as someone who threw himself into whatever he did—studies, relationships, sports, and his faith.

In 1948, Jim felt called to minister in South America. After college graduation, he worked to make that dream a reality and eventually moved to Ecuador with his wife and four other missionary couples. Jim took the same enthusiastic and aggressive approach to his mission work, and the five men endeavored to reach a violent Indian tribe in the interior of that country.

The work seemed to be going well; they were building trust with the

Indians. But suddenly, on January 8, 1956, the airwaves were filled with news that all five men had been murdered by the people they had been trying to reach. Most couldn't understand the dedication and drive of these young men and the "waste" of their lives.

Years earlier, Jim had determined to go wherever God would lead him, to share the gospel, no matter what the cost. In his journal he had written, "Consume my life, my God, for it is [yours]. I seek not a long life, but a full one, like you, Lord Jesus." Jim knew the one for whom he was living, and nothing else mattered. His life was short but full as he ran for Christ.

The Race

Because we are living for our audience of one, like Jim Elliot we should work hard and with enthusiasm—that is, we should pick up the pace, increase our speed. Some do as little as possible, just enough to get by in school, on the job, in relationships, even in church. That would be like a runner entering a "race" and then simply running at a slow jog from start to finish. And sadly, some people live that way (even some Christians), simply coasting through life, playing it safe.

Picking up the pace means loving our families (home), doing our jobs well and doing more than we're asked (work), serving our neighbors and needy people we know (community), volunteering and using our spiritual gifts (church), and praying for and financially supporting believers and ministries in other countries (world).

And it means doing all this with *joy*, regardless of how others respond.

The Result

God doesn't expect you to "win" or to do better than anyone else. He just wants your best in every arena, for you to push for a personal record. And that's because you're running "for the Lord rather than for people." Jim Elliot also said, "He is no fool who gives what he cannot keep to gain that which he cannot lose."

So what's holding you back? Now is the time in your race to increase your speed.

My Story

I've never considered myself to be a "runner," even though at this point I've been running for more than half of my adult life. When I began running at the urging of a good friend (mostly to keep my weight down when my metabolism slowed), we were in northern Wisconsin in July and running on a paved road. We would run between two telephone poles and then walk between the next two, and so on—not too tough and not too long. Eventually my running workout increased to a mile. But I never enjoyed it; at that time, running was simply a means to an end.

Then my wife, daughter, and I moved from the Chicago suburbs to the New Orleans area, where I was able to continue running outside. That spring, a friend suggested running in a 5K race in our town. Hmmm—3.1 miles was a stretch for me, but I agreed and began running with that friend. He would usually leave me in the dust or slow his pace to run with me. In either case, he never seemed very tired after our runs, while I was gasping for breath. But I felt stronger each time out.

On race day, we walked to the start and made plans to meet afterward, assuming that my friend would finish way ahead of me. At the starting gun, we took off and ran together in the middle of the pack. I had decided to let him go on when he wanted and to run at my own pace—I wouldn't try to keep up. But we were still together at the end of the first mile, and surprisingly, I was feeling good. So I increased my speed. At about that time, I lost track of my running partner, but I continued on at the faster pace. I actually had enough energy at the end to sprint (if my speed

could be called a "sprint") to the finish. Cooling down,
I looked for my friend among the couple hundred runners.
Eventually we connected and discovered that I had finished
well ahead of him. My "runner" friend was shocked at my
success and kept shaking his head, wondering how that could
have happened.

It's a mystery to me, too. But that race taught me
several valuable lessons . . . about running my own race
at my own pace, about running smart—starting slow and
picking up the pace—and about doing my best and letting
the results take care of themselves. I remembered those
lessons in future races, especially marathons. Now if I
would only apply them to life . . .

Dave

Think It Through

1. What is your normal running pace (minutes/mile)? What do you do to pick up the pace (exert more energy, lengthen your stride, etc.)?
2. In which areas of life do you tend to coast, doing just enough to get by? Why?
3. How would your life change if you lived as if God were your audience and your coach, watching every step?
4. What are a few ways that you can pick up the pace spiritually?

On Running

How does imagery help me when I'm running?

Imagery is simply the mental rehearsal of a performance or practice prior to participation in the activity, creating an experience in your mind. Imagery with running will help you prepare your body for a practice or race. Imagining that you are engaging in running actually causes a small reaction in your imagery-used muscles. Imagery also acts as a mental blueprint, helping you plan what you should do when running. And this practice can increase your confidence and concentration. Overall, imagery can help you build confidence, practice your running form, improve your concentration, and control your emotional responses.

JOURNAL

_____

_____

_____

_____

_____

RUNNING LOG

	TIME	DISTANCE	WEATHER	NOTES
DAY 1				
DAY 2				
DAY 3				
DAY 4				
DAY 5				

INCREASE YOUR SPEED

Some runners who seem to be coasting or taking it easy aren't lazy; they simply are afraid to run faster, thinking they won't have the energy or endurance to continue very long or to finish. But if we've planned well, geared up, trained the right way, and started slow, we should have confidence in our ability to perform at this point in the race. In addition to helping runners build endurance, another reason for including at least one run of eighteen or twenty miles in a marathon training schedule is to build confidence. Knowing that we ran *that* far should help us believe we can run just a 10K farther and finish. It's a matter of faith, trusting in our preparation and what we know about ourselves and running a marathon.

The Bible talks a lot about faith. Here's a familiar example: "Trust in the LORD with all your heart; do not depend on your own understanding. Seek his will in all you do, and he will show you which path to take" (Proverbs 3:5-6).

Trusting in God means depending on his wisdom and strength, not our own. It means asking him what he wants us to do ("seek his will"), and when he shows us, doing it.

That's what David did. And after God rescued him from his enemies and from Saul, he sang, "In your strength I can crush an army; with my God I can scale any wall" (2 Samuel 22:30).

We run—we live—in God's strength, trusting him in every stride.

The Runner

Jesus told a story about a man and three servants. About to leave on a long trip, the man entrusted three servants with bags of silver: five, two, and one, respectively. The servant with five bags invested them and earned five more—100 percent increase. The servant with two bags also doubled the amount through his investments. But the one with a single bag buried the master's money in the ground. When the master returned from his trip, he called together the servants to see how they had handled his money. For the first and second men, he had nothing but praise: "Well done, my good and faithful servant. You have been faithful in handling this small amount, so now I will give you many more responsibilities. Let's celebrate together!" (Matthew 25:21, 23). But here's what happened with the other man:

> The servant with the one bag of silver came and said, "Master, I knew you were a harsh man, harvesting crops you didn't plant and gathering crops you didn't cultivate. I was afraid I would lose your money, so I hid it in the earth. Look, here is your money back."
>
> But the master replied, "You wicked and lazy servant! If you knew I harvested crops I didn't plant and gathered crops I didn't cultivate, why didn't you deposit my money in the bank? At least I could have gotten some interest on it." (MATTHEW 25:24-27)

The master was angry with this man because he was only thinking of himself and making excuses. Because of fear, that man was playing it safe.

Holding back is how many people run. It's also how many people live.

The Race

The third servant was well aware of the risks involved. That's why he buried the money—out of fear of failure. His focus on himself and his predicament caused him to forget about his master.

Living by faith often involves sacrifice and pain and always involves risk. But we do what God wants because we know and trust him—we follow his paths and rely on his strength.

The Result

Saying that we trust God is easy; living it out takes commitment. James wrote, "What good is it, dear brothers and sisters, if you say you have faith but don't show it by your actions? . . . Faith by itself isn't enough. Unless it produces good deeds, it is dead and useless" (James 2:14, 17).

God wants us to live without fear, to run with faith.

Increase your speed!

My Story

Conquering the dark, unknown morning while wearing running shoes frightened my husband more than I ever understood. Not that he feared the potential for hidden dangers in the shadows. But his fear of exchanging cozy, warm blankets for sweats and layered running shirts made our goal of running a race together a fight between newlywed devotion and a natural inclination to sleep in.

Running a 5K together topped our list of goals to complete within five years of marriage. I had brought quite a collection of race T-shirts into our new home, but Walter had yet to earn a single one, and I couldn't wait to be there with him when we crossed that finish

line together. Because I knew his feet hadn't run more
than a half mile in years, however, I also understood we
had much training to do before the upcoming Jingle Bell
Run two weeks before Thanksgiving.

I naturally pop out of bed, usually with a smile on my
face, hours before I need to be anywhere. Running in the
morning fills my energy tank for the day like nothing else
does. Crisp air, the intermittent whooshing of passing
cars, and the warming up of my legs as they loosen and
move in the familiar pounding pattern—I love it. That
time talking to God, often out loud, clears clutter out
of my mind while my heart pumps faster and harder.

Despite becoming one with my husband through our
wedding vows, I soon learned my running passion was
not contagious. If we planned to cross the finish line
together, I had work to do beyond willing my own feet to
move: pep talks, encouraging words, picking his running
clothes out of the dresser—everything short of tying his
shoelaces for him. After all, he needed to make at least
one choice to participate in his training schedule.

For over a month, I led my husband down our street
and across the local university campus for morning "death
marches," as he so fondly refers to them now. For thirty
minutes each morning, I became a cheerleader, an encourager,
and a storyteller. Sometimes I forced myself to look
straight ahead to avoid noticing the scowls he gave me, and
other times I dodged grumpy words reprimanding me for being
too cheerful so early on a frosty morning.

Training complete, we arrived at race day prepared to run
3.106 miles together. While laughing at some of the crazy
costumes competitors in the annual contest wore, I rehearsed
encouraging words and contemplated if I could possibly carry
my husband across the finish line if necessary.

Mostly, I relished that we were doing it—my husband
and I running a race together! Through our mutual sweat
and pain, we were about to accomplish something together
just as we planned.

The gun blasted and changed everything. My sweet non-runner honey almost left me behind from the start!

We raced past beautiful homes and down the local running trail. And then I saw the back of my husband's navy blue running shirt as he pushed past me and closed in on the finish line. After a quick discussion about his intentions, I realized he really could do it. Maybe I hadn't seen his best running face when he rolled out of bed at 5:00 a.m. to accompany me around the neighborhood. But he intended to show me now that the moment counted.

Crossing that finish line almost a minute behind my husband, I was never more happy to have been beaten by anyone. He had found his own motivation somewhere inside, and it didn't depend on my cheery words.

And so we began our married life together wearing our Jingle Bell T-shirts with pride and having accomplished our goal of running a 5K together.

Angie

Think It Through

1. When have you seen an athlete or a team playing tentatively, with fear, playing not to lose instead of to win? What happened?
2. What keeps believers from picking up the pace in their Christian lives, from taking risks for Christ?
3. What are your biggest fears in living by faith?
4. What can you do to increase your trust in God, to rely more on his strength?

On Running

What are tips for imagery?

To get the most out of imagery, begin by finding the proper setting—a place where you won't be interrupted or distracted. Be sure to have a positive focus during this experience. Stay relaxed, and with a sense of relaxed concentration, close your eyes and picture yourself running the race. Be sure to set realistic expectations, that is, don't imagine yourself running as fast as the Olympic champion; focus on *your* strengths and performance. Make your image as vivid and controllable as possible, and do it in real time.

JOURNAL

_____

_____

_____

_____

_____

RUNNING LOG

	TIME	DISTANCE	WEATHER	NOTES
DAY 1				
DAY 2				
DAY 3				
DAY 4				
DAY 5				

FIND A RHYTHM

After runners hit their stride in a long race, they try to find a comfortable running rhythm and maintain that pace for several miles.

Say, for example, someone knows he can run consistently and steadily at a nine-minute-per-mile pace. If he were able to do that for the full 26.2 miles, he would have a time just under four hours—a goal for many marathoners. To reach that goal, then, his strategy should be to run the first five miles at about ten minutes per mile. Then, in picking up the pace and finding his rhythm, he should try to run the next ten miles or so at about eight and a half minutes per mile. If he is able to do this, at the end of fifteen miles, he will have spent two hours and fifteen minutes. So to reach that four-hour goal, he would have to run the last 11.2 miles in under one hour and forty-five minutes, averaging 9.37 minutes per mile—very doable. And if he's feeling good—and the weather cooperates—he may be able to do even better.

The key to making this work is to find that running sweet spot or groove, where running seems almost effortless and the miles roll by. To get to this place, to be able to find a good running rhythm, the runner must have:

- put in the miles to get in shape;
- developed an efficient, fluid running style;
- geared up right, especially the shoes;
- started off slowly, saving the physical reserves;
- and taken fluids early for the body to use later—all points we have covered in previous weeks.

In life, this feels much like those middle, productive years, when we are able to use most effectively our talents and abilities for the Kingdom. Paul told the church in Ephesus, "This will continue until we all come to such unity in our faith and knowledge of God's Son that we will be mature in the Lord, measuring up to the full and complete standard of Christ" (Ephesians 4:13).

Paul had just discussed the role of spiritual gifts in the church, explaining how all the members of the body of Christ work together. (We touched on this in Week 7.) When they begin to hit their stride, they "continue" working together in unity.

The Runner

Now almost thirty, Emma's walk with Christ began in high school when she went with a friend to an event put on by Campus Life, a Christian group with the reputation of being crazy fun. She enjoyed herself, met some new kids, and even put up with the short talk at the end about Jesus. Emma became a regular to the group, and a few months later, she gave her life to Christ.

Emma's life began to change as she got into a small-group Bible study and connected with a church. After high school, Emma continued to grow in her faith in college, where she became a leader in InterVarsity. And that's where she met Dan. Today, seven years into their marriage and with two small children, Emma and Dan are serious about their faith, especially about being Christian parents. They love their church, but between work and the kids, they haven't plugged in anywhere except for a small group of other young couples.

That began to change for Emma one Sunday after listening to a sermon on Ephesians 4. Looking back on her spiritual history, Emma realized that she had been a recipient of so much from God through his people—Campus Life and InterVarsity staff, Christian friends, teachers, pastors, small-group leaders—but she hadn't done much. Even though she was busy as a mom, Emma felt she had to start giving back, using her gifts in the church and community. So she began by signing up to teach Sunday school. She also began attending a women's Bible study, where she became a small-group leader. She knows that's just a start and is looking for more opportunities to serve.

The Race

Emma has been prepared and has warmed up, and now she's starting slow. But soon she'll pick up the pace, find her "running rhythm," and, God willing, actively use her gifts until she's limited by health or other circumstances.

That's the way the church is supposed to work—believers using their gifts and working together. When this happens, Paul says:

Then we will no longer be immature like children. We won't be tossed and blown about by every wind of new teaching. We will not be influenced when people try to trick us with lies so clever they sound like the truth. Instead, we will speak the truth in love, growing in every way more and more like Christ, who is the head of his body, the church. He makes the whole body fit together perfectly. As each part does its own special work, it helps the other parts grow, so that the whole body is healthy and growing and full of love. (EPHESIANS 4:14-16)

That sounds like a whole church finding a rhythm.

The Result

As with runners, no two Christians are identical—each one is a unique blend of physical, personality, and emotional traits and special talents, abilities, and spiritual gifts. And we're all at a different place in life's race—some just beginning and others nearing the finish. That's why we need each other and to serve together, each person being a good servant (like the ones we looked at last week) investing gifts for the Master. And along the route we'll "strengthen those who have tired hands, and encourage those who have weak knees" (Isaiah 35:3).

My Story

I'm not sure I have ever experienced the "runner's high"—
a feeling of euphoria, a result of the body releasing
endorphins during strenuous activity. I guess the closest
I came was during my second marathon. My first marathon
was extremely tough and totally different . . . but that's
another story.

In this one, the weather was great—thirty-seven
degrees at the start, with a slight breeze to our backs.
I began with a friend, and we ran slowly at the start,
not getting caught up in the excitement or worrying about
anyone passing us. After five miles or so, I felt strong
and increased my speed. My pace, however, was too fast for
my buddy, who began to struggle and encouraged me to go
on, so I did. And that's when I seemed to find my rhythm,
where I felt as if I could run forever (I know that's
impossible, but bear with me here).

I've heard basketball players talk about being "in the
zone" when they can't miss and other athletes being "in
the groove," and that's what I compare my "runner's high"
to. I just know that I was able to keep that pace for about
ten miles, and I set my personal record (and it still is).

I find that pattern in other areas of life—working,
playing, and especially serving. I've learned that I need

to take advantage of those times when conditions are right
and I have energy, strength, and other resources and can
make a difference. God expects me to use my gifts for his
glory, and right now I'm in the groove.

Frank

Think It Through

1. In a long run, when do you feel your best, as if you could run forever? How did you discover your running rhythm?
2. How have you been prepared for ministry? What have you done to "warm up" and "start slow"?
3. What special talents, abilities, and spiritual gifts do you bring to the body of Christ?
4. What can you do to find your rhythm in ministry?

On Running

What is flow, and why is it important?

Flow is a holistic sensation when people feel they are totally caught up in an activity, as if they are on automatic pilot. The essential elements of flow are complete absorption in the activity, a merging of action and awareness, a loss of self-consciousness, and a sense of control. The goals or rewards external to the activity aren't relevant at this time, and it is an effortless moment. In order to sense flow, you need confidence, positive thinking, and a high level of motivation. Flow is important because it can help you to feel relaxed, control anxiety, and enjoy what you are doing. Basically, flow is finding your rhythm.

JOURNAL

_____

_____

_____

_____

RUNNING LOG

	TIME	DISTANCE	WEATHER	NOTES
DAY 1				
DAY 2				
DAY 3				
DAY 4				
DAY 5				

FIND A RHYTHM

The running rhythm varies with each runner. Some seem to be born runners—with small, light, long strides and great lung capacity, they almost glide on the track. At the other end of the spectrum come the heavyweights, the over-six-feet-tall and over-two-hundred-pounds guys who seem to lumber along the route—yet both finish and do their best. Every marathon produces runners-who-shouldn't-be-runners stories: an octogenarian, a cancer survivor, a veteran on prosthetics, even a blind competitor. Each of these men and women finds his or her respective rhythm and runs the race, often serving as an example and motivation for others.

Christ's church is marked by variety as well—believers of every shape, age, size, social group, ethnic background, and personal challenge. Yet we come together in local churches and use our unique gifts to minister and serve; we run the race together. And in his grace, God uses some of the least likely to succeed as his choice servants. As Paul reminded the Christians in Corinth:

Remember, dear brothers and sisters, that few of you were wise in the world's eyes or powerful or wealthy when God called you.

Instead, God chose things the world considers foolish in order to shame those who think they are wise. And he chose things that are powerless to shame those who are powerful. God chose things despised by the world, things counted as nothing at all, and used them to bring to nothing what the world considers important.
(1 CORINTHIANS 1:26-28)

Each person needs to choose his or her own pace (Week 21) and find his or her *own* rhythm.

The Runner

Alex was a decent athlete, having played a wide variety of sports growing up, including stints on the high school football and basketball teams. He even played college football. But he never saw himself as a long-distance runner. As Alex aged and his metabolism slowed, he thought he ought to take up jogging for health reasons. Running seemed easy enough—it was faster than walking and didn't require a heavy financial investment. So Alex started slow and over several months worked up to running five miles. And that was a big deal for him.

Alex would hear about marathons, especially the one held annually in his city, but he never seriously considered running in one—that was way beyond his comfort level. Then one day he reconnected with an old friend, Pat. In the course of their conversation, Pat mentioned that he had become a runner (surprising Alex, because Pat was built like a fireplug) and that he had finished a marathon (*shocking* because Pat had lost a knee cap in a sledding accident years ago). After their conversation, Alex thought, *Hmmm—if Pat can run a marathon, I ought to be able to*. About a month later, the sports section reported the results of his city's race and featured a story about a man with no feet—just stumps in socks and shoes—who had finished.

That did it. With both of those men serving as examples, Alex decided to train for next year's race. If they could do it, he could. And he did.

The Race

Alex found inspiration and motivation through what Pat and the man with no feet had accomplished. Alex, in turn, has motivated others through his example. None of those men are world-class runners—far from it. Each one has his own running rhythm and runs his unique race.

In the same way, we can inspire and motivate others by how we run the Christian race, by how we live and serve, even though by the world's standards we aren't "powerful," "wealthy," "wise," or "important." Paul knew that was true. That's why he said, "You should imitate me, just as I imitate Christ" (1 Corinthians 11:1).

The Result

If you ever think you're underqualified or too unimportant to be used by God, remember 1 Corinthians 1:28: "God chose things despised by the world, things counted as nothing at all, and used them to bring to nothing what the world considers important." God will use you to further his Kingdom and to motivate others to do the same.

Understanding that you have a special role to play in Christ's Kingdom, find your spiritual service rhythm and use your gifts for God's glory.

My Story

I have never been one to spend much time running around a track for exercise. And I don't know if I have ever used a treadmill. For me, running is not just a way to stay fit but a chance to explore, to experience the sights, smells, sounds, and climate around me.

I've run on pleasant spring days. I've run through rain, through snow, and in humidity so thick I almost had to grow gills to breathe in the air. The exciting fact is that no two outings are the same. Something is different every time—weather, scenery, people (or animals) I meet along the way.

I've had opportunities to run in different places around the world, too. I've plodded along the flat, straight farm roads of the low country in South Carolina. I've taken in the salty sea air along the coast of Mozambique. I've run up and down the hilly streets of Jerusalem (in the new city). I've jogged past cafés in Spain. I've stared in awe at the majestic mountain peaks in British Columbia. I've enjoyed the brilliant reds and yellows of a New England fall while jogging in New Hampshire.

Of all the places I've run, my favorite is the farmlands of Centenary, Zimbabwe. My parents lived and ministered there during my college years, and I would visit during my summer or Christmas breaks. I remember setting off along the small, winding roads early in the morning at sunrise. The tall blonde grass hung over the edges of the lane, and the hills (kopjes) stood silhouetted against the brightening sky. I would pass villages and the intoxicating smell of cooking fires and the cheerful chatter of grandmothers preparing breakfast. On most mornings I would greet children on their way to school, and sometimes they would run along with me for a while. Then there were the farm laborers harvesting the tobacco crop. And every morning the soothing sound of the laughing dove was medicine for my soul.

In the late afternoons I would go down to the farm compound and play an exhausting game of soccer with the farm workers. We would play on that dusty field until the sun sank below the horizon and we could barely make out the shape of the ball. The next morning I'd hit the road again. There I was in the middle of Africa—out of my element yet at the same time never more in it.

What a gift that God allows us to experience the wonders of his creation each day. And I feel I'm able to take it in even more when I'm out running.

Mark

Think It Through

1. Who are some people who surprised you by finishing a marathon? Why were you surprised?
2. Who has surprised you by how God has used them in ministry? Why were you surprised?
3. In what ways is your spiritual running rhythm unique for you? What gifts are you using for God's glory?
4. Who do you think might be inspired and motivated by seeing how God is using you?

On Running

Why does my heart rate increase when I run?

Heart rate is determined by the amount of blood pushed through the body. Blood carries the needed oxygen for your muscles and brain to function. When you run, your muscles are doing more work and need more oxygen. As your breathing increases to get more oxygen, your heart rate increases in order to move blood more quickly to the needed muscles.

JOURNAL

_____

_____

_____

_____

_____

_____

_____

_____

_____

_____

RUNNING LOG

	TIME	DISTANCE	WEATHER	NOTES
DAY 1				
DAY 2				
DAY 3				
DAY 4				
DAY 5				

BEWARE OF COMPARE

By definition, a "race" is a competition in which a winner is determined. Runners on high school and university cross-country teams compete regularly against other schools and individuals. The object of those races should be to win while doing one's best. Unfortunately, in many athletic contests, winning becomes most important and is achieved by cheating or by pulling down the opponent.

For most runners, especially those not on interscholastic teams, the real competition is against the clock as they strain to reach a personal record. That's how it should work in amateur long-distance races. Often, however, runners compare themselves to other runners and try to "beat" them, especially in the middle part of the race when they're running well and feeling good.

The urge to run faster in order to pass other runners can be a trap, pulling us off our running plan and racing pace. Comparing ourselves to other runners can also be deceptive and harmful. For example, we can think we're doing well because we're passing so many, when in fact our pace is slow. Or trying to stay with faster runners can throw us off stride or cause us to deplete our reserves prematurely. Each person should be disciplined and run his or her own race—no one else's.

Comparisons come easy—we make them constantly, measuring ourselves against how others perform. Instead, we should concentrate on ourselves, on using the gifts that God has given to *us*, running our own races.

Peter learned this lesson after the Resurrection. Jesus had just given Peter his marching orders, including how Peter would die. Then we read:

> *Peter turned around and saw behind them the disciple Jesus loved—the one who had leaned over to Jesus during supper and asked, "Lord, who will betray you?" Peter asked Jesus, "What about him, Lord?" Jesus replied, "If I want him to remain alive until I return, what is that to you? As for you, follow me."* (JOHN 21:20-22)

Did you catch that? When Peter asked about John, Jesus answered, "What is that to you? As for you, follow me." In other words, "Don't worry about John—focus on yourself and your work for me. You have your own race to run."

The Runner

Jessica was prepared for this half marathon, and the weather was perfect—cool, dry, and overcast. As she walked to her place near the starting line, she spotted an old high school track rival, Lauren, and greeted her. They stood just a few feet apart, and when the starter's gun sounded, both runners took off. Lauren's pace was a little faster than Jessica's, so she pushed a bit to pull even. But then Lauren increased her speed to pull ahead; Jess matched that increase. Soon they were running way too fast for the start . . . and neither one finished.

A natural athlete and very competitive, Jordan had excelled at most of the sports he had tried. And although he had never run competitively, he used the same drive and workout ethic when he became a "runner." After entering a few 10K races, Jordan decided to go for it—the marathon. So he read everything he could on it, got a training schedule, and faithfully put in the miles.

At the start of the race, Jordan was disciplined and ran slower than he thought he could. But he couldn't stand being passed by older or heavier runners—even some women! So he began to increase his speed, choosing a runner in the distance and making his goal to pass him or her. He got so caught up in this process that he blew past the aid stations—after all, think of all the chumps he could pass who were taking time to drink. Jordan cramped up at mile twenty and eventually staggered across the finish line, behind many of those older, heavier, and female competitors.

After the marathon, Seth, Greg, and Sue were limping, rehydrating, and talking about the experience. The three friends had trained together and now had gathered for their ride home. This was the first marathon for each, and all three were thrilled that they had reached their goals—they had finished. Seth's time was four hours and nine minutes; Greg finished in three hours and fifty-four minutes; Sue took almost five hours to complete the course. But they celebrated with and for each other, knowing that each one had done his or her best.

The Race

When we compare ourselves to others and don't measure up, we can begin to think poorly of ourselves and our abilities. Or if we outdo someone else, we can puff up with pride. Or, similar to a child comparing his pile of Christmas presents to a sibling's, we can think, *It's just not fair!* That may have been what was lurking at the edge of Peter's mind when he asked about John. The comparison game only hurts our performance. Instead, we need to hear Jesus' words: "*You follow me.*"

The Result

The Christian life isn't a competition, a contest. God doesn't expect us to do *better* than anyone else . . . just our best for him. Paul told the believers in Galatia, "Pay careful attention to your own work, for then you will get the satisfaction of a job well done, and you won't need to compare yourself to anyone else. For we are each responsible for our own conduct" (Galatians 6:4-5).

Stay focused on running *your* race, regardless of how well or poorly anyone around you is doing.

My Story

My son's seventh-grade student-parent cross-country meet was held on a cold, wet autumn day. Watching my son enjoy success in running brought me true joy. Still an active runner and triathlete, I thought I would humor my son and run alongside the little guy for the 1.5-mile event.

The gun went off, and we all joyfully began the short, competitive run across the plains of the middle school campus. I knew I couldn't keep pace with the number one boy runner, but I was confident that I could stay with my son through the finish line.

As the race went on, my son quietly pulled away from me at the quarter-mile point. I held back, thinking I would simply stay on his tail until the end and then run him down for fun. As the run continued, I figured I had better turn on a little speed at the three-quarter-mile mark to pull him in. So I put the hammer down and worked very hard to draw closer. To my surprise, he had more in the tank than I ever knew and continued to pull away. Giving my best effort, I poured all my adult energy into the final half mile with the expectation to finish in a blaze of glory, albeit behind my boy. Two boys were ahead of my son, and I thought, what the heck, a fourth-place finish behind my boy wouldn't be so bad. After all, I have a lot of excuses. As I continued to drive to the finish line with all the energy I could physically muster, Molly, a seventh-grade girl, came flying by me as if I were jogging and hammered to a strong fourth-place finish.

Dear old dad finished fifth, puzzled, humbled, but happy. My boy was all smiles. The baton had been passed. (Hmmm, and I thought I had at least another year of being the fast guy!)

Don R.

Think It Through

1. Why do we tend to compare ourselves to others in running and other areas of life?
2. In what ways can competition hurt competitors?
3. When have you felt as if you didn't measure up because of someone else's performance?
4. If Jesus were saying to you, "What is that to you? You follow me," what would you think? How would that change the way you live?

On Running

Is it okay to be on a low-carbohydrate diet?

Runners should keep a regular-carbohydrate diet because carbohydrates are the body's main source of energy. After depleting those resources, the body switches to using fat. That sounds great for people losing weight; however, fats take longer to break down and provide energy. Most likely, without carbohydrates you wouldn't have enough energy for a good run that would help you burn more calories. This doesn't mean you should switch to a high-carbohydrate diet; just try to maintain a regular-carbohydrate diet.

JOURNAL

_____

_____

_____

_____

_____

RUNNING LOG

	TIME	DISTANCE	WEATHER	NOTES
DAY 1				
DAY 2				
DAY 3				
DAY 4				
DAY 5				

BEWARE OF COMPARE

The other side of comparisons is the fear of what others might think of us. And this fear can cause us to make foolish decisions. Sometimes, for example, we might wear clothes that look great but don't protect us from the elements. Or we might feel pressured by a person or group to do what we shouldn't—the desire to enhance our image overrules our common sense (or spiritual sense).

During this competitive stage of the race, we may think that people (other runners, spectators, race volunteers, etc.) are impressed by how fast we're running, the way we're passing runners, or by our ability to run through pain. Thinking that way can be dangerous for a variety of reasons, not the least of which is safety. We should run our own races and not worry about what others think about how we look, our running style, or our speed.

That's basically the lesson of 1 Corinthians 4:2-4:

A person who is put in charge as a manager must be faithful. As for me, it matters very little how I might be evaluated by you or by any human authority. I don't even trust my own judgment on

this point. My conscience is clear, but that doesn't prove I'm right.
It is the Lord himself who will examine me and decide.

The issue, according to Paul, is *faithfulness,* knowing that God is the only judge of his character and actions who matters. We should live for him, no one else.

The Runner

Hall of Fame college coach Bud Wilkinson was only thirty-one when he became the head football coach at the University of Oklahoma. Over his seventeen years at that university, he amassed an amazing record of 145-29-4, including forty-seven wins in a row, four undefeated seasons, and three national championships. The secret to the success of those teams and for Bud as a coach was simple: The players knew that only one person's evaluation of them mattered—his.

Anyone who has ever competed in sports understands that every contest has potential distractions for the competitors. For example, athletes can play for themselves, to get glory; that motivation is poison for a team. Some may worry about how their teammates are doing and focus on them instead of on their own performance. Some might play to the other team's level and get distracted by the poor or dirty play of their opponents. And, of course, some can play to the fans, perhaps a favorite one or two.

Bud worked hard at getting his athletes to focus on themselves, no one else. His players learned that what the fans saw or what other players, teammates, or opponents did was not important. All that mattered was what *Bud* saw, how *he* evaluated their individual performances.

Bud understood the principle of not comparing ourselves to others.

The Race

God's Word tells us how to live, how to run for him. That should be our only performance standard. Comparing ourselves to anything will only confuse or harm us. We may become prideful, thinking highly of ourselves, as these men referenced by Paul: "Oh, don't worry; we wouldn't dare say that we are as wonderful as these other men who tell you how important they are! But they are only comparing themselves with each other, using themselves as the standard of measurement. How ignorant!" (2 Corinthians 10:12).

Or we may begin to think we're worthless when compared to spiritual or moral elites.

God's message is quite different—he made us, loves us, cheers for us, and is working for our success. We matter to him.

The Result

What does our heavenly Coach want from us? Jesus put it very plainly: "The most important commandment is this: . . . 'You must love the LORD your God with all your heart, all your soul, all your mind, and all your strength.' The second is equally important: 'Love your neighbor as yourself.' No other commandment is greater than these" (Mark 12:29-31).

Run for *him*. Run *his* race. Don't compare.

My Story

I love sports. Not just playing, or even just watching;
I like to analyze and provide my own commentary. Sports
are a part of who I am. I've always been an athlete and
participated in numerous sports, but in college I only
played intramurals and ran to stay in shape. I loved those
activities, but I tended to compare myself to others who
played. Although I wasn't on a college team, I wanted to
prove that I still was an athlete.

During my junior year I started working with the men's
soccer team. As the only female, I felt a desire to
prove myself. That year, I also had my first of two foot
surgeries. So during the summer I trained and finished
the Chicago Triathlon (Olympic distance). I was proud of
my accomplishment but didn't really enjoy myself because

I focused on where I lacked and on the other people (especially my friends) who finished ahead of me. Instead, I should have been happy for how I had done, thanking God for giving me the ability to participate and finish.

The summer after I graduated (and after another foot surgery), I began training for the Chicago Marathon. This time I took a different approach. I decided to run for myself, not to please or beat anyone else. I began to train and signed up for the race without telling anyone. I eventually told my dad so that he could run one more marathon, this time with his daughter. Here and there people would know I was training, but I worked hard to keep it a secret. Why? Because I didn't want the attention—I wasn't trying to prove myself anymore. I didn't want to be compared to anyone. In the end, I loved every second of that marathon.

Comparing ourselves to others is natural and easy, even in our spiritual lives. When we see missionaries or more high-profile Christians, we may feel as if we need to prove that we are good Christians as well. When that happens, we become more concerned about looking good to other believers than about really serving God. But we don't need to prove ourselves to God. He knows us and loves us, imperfections and all. Instead of living for others, we live for Christ, secure in our relationship with our loving Father.

Dana

Think It Through

1. When have you made a foolish decision based on what someone thought of you?

2. In running, how have you compared yourself to others? How have those comparisons made you feel? How did they affect your performance?

3. What does loving God with all your heart, soul, mind, and strength mean to you?

4. If you believed you only had to please God with your actions, how would that affect your choices, thoughts, and lifestyle?

On Running

When should I ramp up to a high carbohydrate diet?

A high-carbohydrate diet is mainly for endurance runners. Anyone planning to run long distances should have plenty of carbohydrates in the diet. That's because the most easily accessible form of energy in the body is glycogen—a form of carbohydrate. Having a high-carbohydrate diet for long-duration exercise (more than four hours), high-intensity/medium-duration exercise (one to two hours), and high-intensity exercise (less than one hour) will maintain your glycogen stores and give you consistent energy throughout your running workout.

JOURNAL

RUNNING LOG

	TIME	DISTANCE	WEATHER	NOTES
DAY 1				
DAY 2				
DAY 3				
DAY 4				
DAY 5				

PUSH AHEAD

In every long-distance race, especially a marathon, most runners experience several stages. We've already discussed the start (the first five miles or so) and the competitive stage (the next ten miles when we increase our speed and find our rhythm). Now we hit the *serious* stage, where we don't feel that great and realize that more than ten miles remain to the finish. But we motor on, gamely putting one foot in front of the other, trying to keep our rhythm and fighting those doubts about whether we'll make it to the end. At this point, concerned with our physical and mental issues, we stop worrying about how we look or how we're doing compared to others. This is the "serious" stage because at this point in the race, few runners are smiling.

The parallel to life is obvious. Young people dash out at the start, full of enthusiasm and energy. Then, as they become involved in career and marriage, climbing the economic and marriage/parenting ladder, they measure their success by how they compare to others in their age and social bracket. They're running fast and feeling good. Before they know it, however (often in their forties and fifties), life begins to beat them up—financial reversals, relational conflicts, career setbacks, physical challenges—and they turn deadly serious. But life, their race, continues.

The writer of Hebrews describes life as a long-distance race, and chapter 12 begins by mentioning a "huge crowd of witnesses." These are people who have successfully finished the race (many described in chapter 11) despite incredible obstacles. That heritage of faith should encourage us and give us hope.

> *Therefore, since we are surrounded by such a huge crowd of witnesses to the life of faith, let us strip off every weight that slows us down, especially the sin that so easily trips us up. And let us run with endurance the race God has set before us. We do this by keeping our eyes on Jesus, the champion who initiates and perfects our faith. Because of the joy awaiting him, he endured the cross, disregarding its shame. Now he is seated in the place of honor beside God's throne. Think of all the hostility he endured from sinful people; then you won't become weary and give up.*
> (HEBREWS 12:1-3)

At this point in life, we need to "run with endurance," stripping down to the basics, remembering these other faithful runners, and "keeping our eyes on Jesus," our champion and leader.

The Runner

During high school, Thom had played sports and had been active in music and drama, so he was pretty well known and had lots of friends. He had been a decent student and had been involved in the campus Christian club as well. So Thom was looking forward to his tenth high school reunion. Since graduation, he had gone to college, where he had played football and had met his future wife. After graduation, Thom had earned his master's degree, gotten married, and started his career with a major corporation. So Thom was eager to let his former classmates know he had done well. But the reunion felt a lot like high school, with people falling into their old cliques and "in-crowd, out-crowd" attitudes, with superficial conversation. Most of the discussions seemed to center on how well everyone was doing, as if they were competing.

The next few reunions (every five years) felt the same. Sure, Thom had a good time connecting with old high school buds, but he always left feeling that everyone was stuck in the past and trying to prove something to each other. So he almost skipped the twenty-fifth-year reunion. But he went and was surprised at the change. Besides everyone seeming much more relaxed, they also were more open and honest about their hurts and struggles. In his circle of friends alone, he heard of divorce, heart attack, serious illness, and the loss of a child. Thom had recently been downsized, and his teenagers were giving him fits—so he had some good conversations about how to deal with those issues. He also connected with a couple of former classmates who had become Christians and were active in their church. They promised to pray for each other. *It's amazing how people get serious and stop playing games when reality hits*, Thom thought.

The Race

Now into their forties, Thom and his former classmates are entering the serious stage of life's marathon. Some are still comparing and competing, but most are beginning to reevaluate their life's trajectory and values. And they're vulnerable and looking for help.

During all of life, we need to remember our purpose and focus on our goal, but during these hard times we feel the need for this more than ever. Some can't deal with life and get tripped up by sin. Others struggle on, feeling discouragement and despair. If we want to run our races well, however, we need to take those steps as directed in Hebrews 12: Strip off those weights (i.e., get rid of those sinful habits and thoughts), stay focused on Christ, and think of all he went through for us.

The Result

If you're at an early life stage, be wise and prepared for this one. If you're in this serious stage, stay focused on Christ and his route for you. Jesus said, "Here on earth you will have many trials and sorrows. But take heart, because I have overcome the world" (John 16:33).

Now that's a promise we can run with!

My Story

For a long time I was so captivated by the mental picture of the "huge crowd of witnesses" watching from the grandstands in Hebrews 12:1 that I didn't really pay much attention to the two required personal responses: stripping off weights (sin) and running with endurance my particular race. I don't think I understood at the deepest level the experience behind those responses until I was in my midtwenties.

As part of a leadership training requirement, I signed up for a wilderness learning seminar that would take me into the Upper Peninsula of Michigan for three weeks of intensive outdoor experiences designed to prepare those who would in turn use the natural environment as the context for ministry with young people. The brochure described training in canoeing, kayaking, ropes, backpacking, and camping and hinted at other exotic experiences. What it didn't emphasize was the philosophy of learning by being. We were not going to be allowed to be outside observers and learners—we would be learning in the laboratory of personal experiences.

I wasn't really prepared for two weeks of daily slogging through the mosquito-infested, swampy, hot Northwoods wearing a seventy-pound backpack—a significant amount of the time in the rain. I'm not very big (lighter back then), and my pack equaled about half my weight. I struggled to carry it, and even the rest stops were miserable because I had to plan how to get the pack back on without causing a scene. One guy on our trip would

pick up his pack with one hand and put it on with no more
difficulty than slipping into a sweater. (I hated him.) I
ran the risk of making a fool of myself each time I tried
to get into the harness without crying out over the open
sores on my shoulders where the chafing had worn away my
skin. This went on for fourteen days.

I don't remember that the carrying ever became easier,
and I lost about ten pounds I didn't have to spare. However,
I did learn some tricks for getting into the pack harness,
and as we consumed our food, the packs got a little lighter.
On the morning of the fifteenth day, we were reminded that
one of our final challenges was a ten-mile run.

We left our backpacks in a truck along with everything
we didn't need to carry for the run. Run? I had struggled
with *trudging* for the last two weeks! As I reluctantly
walked to the starting line in the woods, I felt odd
without the pack. I'd grown accustomed to the weight. But
I really noticed the difference when they sent us on our
way. As I ran, I seemed to be floating. I can't remember a
time when I felt so light! It was as if both a mental and
a physical weight that had been pushing down relentlessly
for days had been lifted from my shoulders. The result of
its sudden removal was buoyancy! Running had never felt
so good! And I understood as never before why I needed
to "strip off every weight that slows us down, especially
the sin that so easily trips us up" if I was ever going to
seriously enjoy and succeed at running "with endurance the
race God has set" for me.

Neil

Think It Through

1. During a long-distance race, what weights have you discarded to
   make running easier? When have you been tripped up or hindered by
   something you were wearing?
2. What signs do you have that you are entering or are in the serious stage
   of your life race?

3. What weights do you need to discard in order to run well?
4. What other steps can you take to "run with endurance" the race God has for you?

On Running

What is carbohydrate loading?

Carbohydrate loading is a way to increase carbohydrate stores prior to a long-distance or difficult race. Runners increase their intake of carbohydrates progressively the week before the race in order to build up energy stores to their fullest. Carbohydrate loading is not beneficial for non-racing runners. It should only be used by those engaging in long-duration or high-intensity/medium-duration exercise. It is mainly used as an ergogenic aid—something to enhance performance.

JOURNAL

_____

_____

_____

_____

RUNNING LOG

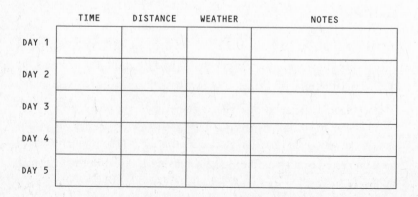

	TIME	DISTANCE	WEATHER	NOTES
DAY 1				
DAY 2				
DAY 3				
DAY 4				
DAY 5				

PUSH AHEAD

During this serious stage of a race, discouragement can set in. Just a few miles earlier, we were feeling good and moving along at the desired pace. But now we're weary in body and spirit. Our legs feel heavy, our breathing is labored, and we know we have a long way to the finish. Doubts nibble at our resolve, and we begin to consider quitting as an option. That's when we need to be mentally and emotionally tough and to dig deep. We've made it this far in our training, and we know we can do it here. We *will* endure to the end.

Making it through this stage of a race and of life takes confidence and resolve, knowing where our strength lies. Centuries ago, the apostle Paul was languishing in prison, awaiting his trial and his eventual execution. Paul didn't know what the future would hold for him, but he knew the one who held his future. So he could write with confidence, "God chose me to be a preacher, an apostle, and a teacher of this Good News. That is why I am suffering here in prison. But I am not ashamed of it, for I know the one in whom I trust, and I am sure that he is able to guard what I have entrusted to him until the day of his return" (2 Timothy 1:11-12).

Paul was confident of his relationship with God. He also knew the source of his strength. Earlier he had written, "This is the secret: Christ lives in you. . . . That's why I work and struggle so hard, depending on Christ's mighty power that works within me" (Colossians 1:27, 29)

The Runner

Melanie was prepared for this race; she really was, having trained for several weeks, following a schedule recommended by a multi-marathon runner. She had run this race by the book, warming up, starting slow, hydrating early, applying Vaseline where needed, and keeping to her planned pace at the appropriate intervals. And she had felt fine . . . until about the mile seventeen marker. And now she was weakening and wondering if she'd make it. Eight miles to go, and she felt like crud. She could almost hear the voices whispering . . .

- "The weather is too warm; no wonder you're sapped!"
- "Hey, you did the best you could, and no one would blame you if you stopped now. Don't kill yourself!"
- "You'll . . . never . . . make . . . it."

But then Melanie remembered what Shelley, another marathon-running friend, had told her—this would happen, but she could make it through. And Melanie thought of Philippians 4:13, a favorite Bible verse and one she had memorized as a kid: "I can do everything through Christ, who gives me strength." She began to repeat it over and over in her head.

Slowly Melanie began to regain her confidence as she called on those spiritual, emotional, and physical reserves. And she ran, one stride after the other and one mile at a time . . . enduring to the end.

The Race

Hardships come in many forms. In running, it might be a leg cramp, a stitch in the side, a spot rubbed raw, overwhelming weariness, or a combination of all of these—but we keep pushing ahead toward our goal. In life, we can experience physical, emotional, relational, mental, financial, and even spiritual tough times. As we struggle along with blurred vision, we may begin to lose hope. Just as Melanie did in her marathon, we need to remember God's promises and rely on his strength to run his race and to run well.

The Result

When you trusted Christ as Savior, the Holy Spirit took up residence in you. So God's "mighty power" is available to you moment by moment—power to change, to endure, to persevere, to resist, to overcome, and to make a difference. Whatever your hardship or challenge, call on those reserves and run in his strength.

My Story

Marathons are 26.2 miles of life-changing excitement, dedicated work, deep determination, and faith that many months of disciplined training will see you to the finish line. It is a choice to train and run. Some will fall away from the challenge as the reality takes shape.

Life's marathons are a different sort. We usually never sign up, the finish line is not really in sight, and yet they, too, can be physically and emotionally grueling. At those times, when things become really hard, we see some fall away who desire an instant miracle with no personal cost.

For me, these life marathons are a process as well. Generally, things will start out feeling comfortable. As the days unfold and the hills become higher, the valleys deeper, the twists and turns may bring no relief or end in sight. This is when I know I must draw upon my faith to keep going. When the desire to endure seems overwhelming, God will bring encouragement. My hope in him provides strength to keep moving forward one step at a time. The days I can't run I

will walk by faith, not by sight. I know there is always a
personal cost and always a reward, yet I won't necessarily
recognize the finish line when I cross it. The process
evolves, and I am forever changed by it.

Becky W.

Think It Through

1. When you've been in the "serious stage" of a race, how have you handled the feelings of discouragement and thoughts of quitting? What kept you going?
2. When have you experienced God's power and strength in your life?
3. What hardships or challenges are you facing right now?
4. What can you do to push through and push forward with hope?

On Running

What causes fatigue?

Fatigue can be caused by any number of factors. During a medium-distance run, the cause can be high amounts of lactic acid (inhibiting the breakdown of glycogen—a type of carbohydrate) and high oxygen debt (not enough oxygen is getting to the muscles). This type of fatigue can take as many as two to three days for recovery. In marathon races, the cause is usually lack of carbohydrates. By consuming carbohydrates during the race, you can reduce fatigue. A carbohydrate diet after a workout will prepare your body for your next workout and keep you from becoming tired early.

JOURNAL

RUNNING LOG

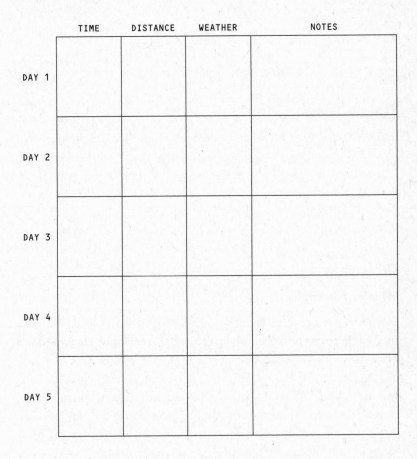

	TIME	DISTANCE	WEATHER	NOTES
DAY 1				
DAY 2				
DAY 3				
DAY 4				
DAY 5				

FUEL UP

Most runners get into the sport because they want to be physically fit—some because of a health scare (the doctor said, "You'd better lose some weight!"), some to prevent health problems, and many just to look good, feel good, and do their best. But exercise is just part of the equation—nutrition is also important. To operate at peak efficiency, our bodies need the right amounts of vitamins, minerals, carbohydrates, proteins, and other food-fuel ingredients—in the right portions. A junk-food diet just won't cut it.

For runners, this means fueling up before, during, and after the race—making sure to be hydrated. And we need to be wise in what and when we eat and drink, especially in a long run such as a marathon. During the start and faster portion of the race, we may not *feel* thirsty and may hate to slow down for a drink at the aid stations. But that's exactly when we should because we'll need that water later. Waiting until mile eighteen when we're depleted and dehydrated will be too late.

Interestingly, the Bible uses drinking to describe aspects of the spiritual life. Peter writes, "Like newborn babies, you must crave pure spiritual milk so that you will grow into a full experience of salvation.

Cry out for this nourishment, now that you have had a taste of the Lord's kindness" (1 Peter 2:2-3).

Just as our physical bodies need milk, our spiritual bodies need God's nourishment, which comes from God and his Word. This food should be so important to us that we "cry out" for it.

The Runner

In the year after his wedding, Devon had put on a few pounds. *Probably from all the good cooking*, he thought. Then he got a promotion at work—great news, except that in his new position he was spending much more time behind a desk, not being very active. So he noticed that he was getting a bit soft around the middle. Devon had always had a big appetite. At six foot five, he could consume great quantities at most meals, and he loved his French fries and wouldn't even try to resist snacks and treats. So gradually he added more weight, especially as his metabolism began to slow.

At first no one noticed because he was a big man. But then his wife and a couple of friends implied that he was getting a bit larger. The friends also suggested that he go with them to the gym or at least try running.

Devon laughed. How could he ever find the time with a small child, the demands of work, and his responsibilities at church? But when he tipped the scale at thirty pounds overweight during his annual physical exam, with high blood pressure and alarming cholesterol numbers, at the urging of his doctor, he decided to do something.

"Gotcha, Doc," Devon told his physician. "I'll start a running program. Right now, I'll probably get winded running a block! But I'll try to work up to running three or four miles every other day or so. Then I can eat anything I want, right?"

"Are you kidding?" the doctor answered. "That would be like continuing to smoke after being diagnosed with lung problems. An exercise program is just part of the solution. An important part to be sure, but you also need to watch the quality and quantity of what you eat."

The Race

Some runners are like Devon, rationalizing bad eating habits with statements like, "Well, I ran today, so I guess another helping won't hurt!" But as the old saying goes, "You are what you eat."

Some Christians act the same way, rationalizing bad spiritual eating habits with statements like, "I went to church, so I'm good with God for this week." Or we might think that reading the "Daily Devotional app" and saying a quick prayer should do the trick. Some may even substitute reading a Christian fiction book or watching a TV evangelist for spending time in Bible study. Certainly church, devotionals, quick prayers, Christian fiction, and religious TV are fine. But they can be like snacking. Our spiritual lives need to be nourished.

Paul writes, "Don't be drunk with wine, because that will ruin your life. Instead, be filled with the Holy Spirit, singing psalms and hymns and spiritual songs among yourselves, and making music to the Lord in your hearts. And give thanks for everything to God the Father in the name of our Lord Jesus Christ" (Ephesians 5:18-20).

Paul's advice: Be careful of what you take in. You were made to run on God, so be filled with his Spirit. And how are we fed spiritually? Through worship individually and with others, praising God for who he is and what he has done for us. Other spiritual nourishment comes from strong Bible teaching and personal Bible study and prayer.

The Result

Consuming the right spiritual food and drink helps us grow in the faith. We become mature and strong, developing our faith muscles. A good spiritual diet builds our endurance, preparing us for the unexpected turns and other trials in the race. We also need to take the right nourishment *during* the race, helping us push on and through to the finish. We need the right fuel to run well and finish strong.

My Story

My first marathon experience was in the fall of 2001.
A recent college graduate with a degree in kinesiology,
I had studied and mapped out *everything* in regard to the
race, including how to prepare mentally, how to eat, and
how to dress.

Knowing what to wear was the easiest part. I dressed
in layers (the starting temperature was below freezing)
and simply removed and threw to the side of the street
anything that was making me hot. Preparing mentally and
nutritionally was more difficult.

I had trained with a water bottle containing half
Gatorade and half water. I knew my intake during training
should be what I would consume during the race. I figured
I probably wouldn't be able to take water and Gatorade at
all the aid stations, so that's why I mixed them. Then,
during the race, I alternated. My first water break was
around mile four or five. Then at the next station I
grabbed Gatorade; the next station water; the next station
Gatorade; and so forth. I also trained using power gel
after learning what gel would be distributed at the race.
I took my first gel around mile twelve (with water, of
course). They handed out a pack around mile eighteen,
but I held on to it and waited until mile twenty-one to
consume it with water. I had trained well, so I knew when
I would need that extra energy—not at mile eighteen.

One of the greatest challenges in a marathon is mental.
I had to stay focused, keep my own pace, and not compare
myself to others. I knew where I would start to feel my
weakest and developed a mental game plan. Around mile
twenty, I started focusing on smaller goals. At each water
station, I told myself to just make it to the next water
station. I continued those small goals until I reached
that finish line.

I fueled and prepared myself mentally and nutritionally,
and at the end of the race, I felt great! Sure, I was

exhausted, but I loved every minute of that run *and* I
never hit the wall—because I learned where to fuel up
nutritionally *and* mentally.

Dana

Think It Through

1. In what ways has running affected what you eat and when? What else caused you to change your diet through the years?
2. When have you substituted spiritual "junk food" or "snacks" for nourishment?
3. Where can you find the spiritual nourishment you need?
4. What changes will you make in your spiritual diet to help you fuel up for your life race? What spiritual food will you consume during your race?

On Running

When should I drink water, and when should I drink a sports drink?

What you drink depends on the length of your workout and the amount you sweat. Generally, if your run is less than one hour, you only need water. In a warm and humid atmosphere, however, when you are sweating a lot, you may need to drink a little bit of a sports drink to replace the electrolytes you lost from your excessive sweating. Of course, if you have trouble drinking a lot of water, try drinking half water/half sports drink to give you some flavor while at the same time replenishing lost fluids.

JOURNAL

_____

_____

_____

_____

_____

RUNNING LOG

	TIME	DISTANCE	WEATHER	NOTES
DAY 1				
DAY 2				
DAY 3				
DAY 4				
DAY 5				

FUEL UP

We've been discussing "fuel," the importance of feeding our bodies and spirits with the right foods, being well fed and nourished for the race. We have seen that monitoring our consumption is vital, but the timing of our intake is also important. The word *fuel* is familiar because we make regular trips to the gas station. A car's fuel supply only lasts for a limited number of miles. So when the dashboard gauge tells us the tank is almost empty, we drive to the station and fill it again.

We also understand the importance of fueling up on a regular basis physically. Imagine someone going to the local all-you-can-eat buffet, pigging out, and then announcing, "Well, that ought to hold me over for another week!" Not a healthy choice—our bodies weren't meant to operate that way. Instead, we take daily, scheduled breaks to eat. Usually that means breakfast, lunch, and dinner.

Runners know that they need to refuel as they go, especially during a long-distance race—those aid stations are regularly spaced for a reason. We don't drink a gallon of water at the beginning of the marathon and think that'll take care of our hydration needs. (We'd sure slosh around when we tried to run.)

So why do we think we can get away with that approach to spiritual fuel? Some people attend church twice a year—on Christmas and Easter—and think that's all they need. Even people who worship almost every weekend can make the mistake of thinking one service will take care of them for the week. We need *daily* nourishment.

David certainly knew this. Listen to the words of his song of praise: "Let the whole earth sing to the LORD! Each day proclaim the good news that he saves" (1 Chronicles 16:23).

And the psalm writer adds, "Each day the LORD pours his unfailing love upon me, and through each night I sing his songs, praying to God who gives me life" (Psalm 42:8).

Did you catch that? "Each day proclaim the good news," "each night" sing songs and pray.

The Runner

Now in her thirties, Pilar has gone to church for as long as she can remember. For Sunday school, she dutifully memorized Bible verses, the Ten Commandments, books of the Bible, and the Lord's Prayer. The easiest of those was the Lord's Prayer because the congregation repeated it together in almost every worship service. So Pilar would recite it along with everyone else, with eyes closed, of course, but not really think much about what she was "praying." But that all changed when the pastor began preaching through Matthew 6:9-13. One Sunday in particular stands out to Pilar—when the sermon highlighted the phrase "give us this day our daily bread." He also turned to Luke 11:3 and read from the New Living Translation: "Give us each day the food we need."

Pilar figured she knew what that phrase meant until the pastor said something like, "*Bread*, as we usually quote from the King James Version, refers to food in general, but it can also mean spiritual food. Also, the Greek word translated 'daily' is an unusual word that occurs only in this prayer in these two places in the New Testament. Using this word reveals that God provides *daily* food, so believers do not need to worry from one day to the next. We cannot store it up and then cut off communication with God. And we dare not be self-satisfied. Instead, we should continually depend on God, day to day."

After that, Pilar knew what she had to do. She went home, found her Bible and a blank notebook to use as a journal, and put them on the coffee table in the living room. Then she prayed, "Father, please give me each day the spiritual nourishment I need. From now on, I will begin each morning with you. Feed me."

The Race

Pilar had discovered how to fuel up for her race.

Jeremiah also learned this lesson. He is called the weeping prophet because he had to continually give bad news about his beloved nation to the king and the people—what a tough marathon! Yet Jeremiah faithfully served God through it all. Tucked away in his book Lamentations, Jeremiah wrote the following lines that you probably remember from a classic hymn: "Great is his faithfulness; his mercies begin afresh each morning" (Lamentations 3:23). Despite all his troubles and trials, Jeremiah could *daily* thank God for being for him and with him. The fuel of God's presence and power gave him strength and courage to keep going.

The Result

God supplies "daily food" as we spend time with him. He is faithful and will supply nourishment "afresh"—but you will need to take it in. Every day feast on his Word, tell him your needs, listen, worship, and declare the Good News. Fuel up . . . and keep running.

My Story

The more years I devote to running, the more adept I become at dressing appropriately for my runs as dictated by changes in the weather or the type of surface on which I'm running. As the heat of summer subsides, I find myself putting away the shorts and the tank tops in favor of running tights and long-sleeve Dri-Fit shirts. I also don a cap with a built-in flashlight on those afternoons when the sun goes to bed by four o'clock. As winter approaches, the fleece comes out of the closet, along with the Yaktrax for icy trail running and perhaps even a face mask to protect my skin from the bitter cold.

This cycle of changing running gear reminds me of how often life can change and how God helps us adjust to the changes. Some life changes are positive, but others, such as the death of a loved one, financial pressures, illness, and job loss, are not so welcome. Despite life's ups and downs, I am comforted when I remember that Jesus is the same yesterday, today, and forever. While I'm out there running ragged trying to cope with the curves in the road and the rocky trails, I am blessed to know I can lean on the one who always travels the same road and is right there beside me no matter how high the mountain or low the valley.

Becky B.

Think It Through

1. What food and drink do you take to help you in long runs and races?
2. Where do you usually obtain your spiritual fuel? How often do you use those resources?
3. How have your spiritual "feeding habits" changed over the past few years?
4. What can you do on a daily basis to fuel up spiritually?

On Running

Meal Timing

PRE-EXERCISE MEAL:
Eat three to five hours beforehand. The amount doesn't really matter; you don't want an insulin response before running (three to ten minutes

before will cause an insulin response). The food you eat, specifically carbohydrates, replenishes your glycogen stores in your muscles so you have the energy you need to run. You don't want to experiment with when you eat your meal, or what you eat, right before a race or competition—stick with what you know. Experiment only during training.

DURING EXERCISE:
Taking carbohydrate solutions for workouts less than sixty minutes is not very beneficial. For longer events, take some type of carbohydrate solution every fifteen minutes.

AFTER EXERCISE:
The first two hours are crucial. Within the first four hours, consume 1.5 grams of carbohydrates per kilogram of body weight for glycogen replenishment. Sports drinks and gels are *very* beneficial. A small amount of protein with carbohydrates will help glycogen replenishment even more. High amounts of carbohydrates produce more power than low amounts over weeks of training.

JOURNAL

_____

_____

_____

_____

_____

_____

_____

_____

_____

RUNNING LOG

	TIME	DISTANCE	WEATHER	NOTES
DAY 1				
DAY 2				
DAY 3				
DAY 4				
DAY 5				

ENJOY THE JOURNEY

Because we set goals and have an ultimate purpose for running, we can easily make each run and race simply a means to an end, something we do or endure in order to achieve something else. That's fine, of course, but in the process we can miss out on a lot. And running can become drudgery, something we *have* to do, just like swallowing bitter medicine that the doctor ordered. Soon we can dread lacing up the shoes and going out for a run. In the process, we can miss sights, sounds, and valuable life lessons.

A few millennia ago, overwhelmed by the beauty of creation, David wrote:

> When I look at the night sky and see the work of your fingers—
> the moon and the stars you set in place—what are mere mortals
> that you should think about them, human beings that you should
> care for them? Yet you made them only a little lower than God
> and crowned them with glory and honor. You gave them charge of
> everything you made, putting all things under their authority—
> the flocks and the herds and all the wild animals, the birds in

the sky, the fish in the sea, and everything that swims the ocean currents. O LORD, our Lord, your majestic name fills the earth!
(PSALM 8:3-9)

Whether David was running, walking, or just sitting and gazing toward the heavens, he saw God and just had to break into praise. To do that, he had to be looking and aware.

The Runner

All of Luke's relatives, friends, and coworkers knew one truth about him—he was *driven*. Definitely a type A personality, Luke was totally goal oriented, and he dedicated himself to reaching those goals. As a student, he had studied hard to be at the top of his class. In his career, he was moving quickly up the corporate ladder. When he joined a local running club, he soon became the one pushing the others. He approached his volunteer efforts in the community and church with the same driven gusto. And everyone knew if they wanted something done—well and quickly—they should give it to Luke. Everything he did, no matter how difficult or distasteful, was a means to an end, a way to achieve what he wanted.

But Luke began to change when he experienced a miracle—the birth of his first child. For years, he and Joanne had prayed for a baby and had tried every medical procedure, with no positive results. And they were way down the list for adoption. They hadn't been able to achieve their goal of parenthood . . . until that moment of their son's birth.

As he and Joanne held little Seth in the hospital, time seemed to slow to a crawl while they marveled at God's amazing work in their arms. And when they brought him home, they treasured every minute with him, even the night feedings. During those times, as Luke gently tried to rock Seth back to sleep, he talked to God and began to reorder his priorities. And during his daily Bible readings, God opened his eyes to the other miracles in his life.

Is Luke still a hardworking, goal-oriented man? Sure. And he still runs at least three miles a day. But he's much more relaxed and seems to be having fun. He has begun to enjoy the journey.

The Race

Like runners who don't enjoy running and run only for the goal, many people (Christians included) miss the joy of living. For example, they only work for the paycheck. They may hate the job and endure the work, but they put in their eight hours a day. Also, they devote a good chunk of each day to sleep, probably seven or eight hours every night. So that leaves only eight more hours. Then subtract drive time, relational conflicts, and unpleasant tasks at home, and—do the math—we can see that they're living but not enjoying life very much. They certainly aren't taking time to see God around them.

But he's there, in nature, people, conversations, and circumstances. And God has placed us where we are for a reason.

Tucked into a discussion with the Corinthians about eating certain foods, Paul drops this gem: "So whether you eat or drink, or whatever you do, do it all for the glory of God" (1 Corinthians 10:31).

Did you catch that? He said, "Whatever you do, do it all for the glory of God." The "whatever" includes working, playing, relating, and running.

The Result

Running for God's glory can be difficult when you're not feeling good already, when bad weather hits, or when you're at the serious section of a long-distance run. And it can be even tougher in other difficult times in life. But that's when we need to look up "at the night sky" and look around and see God and run for him.

So instead of simply putting up with school, work, and obligations, enjoy the journey, doing *everything* for God's glory.

My Story

The thing I love about running is the way it enables me to know a place, to see the scenes I wouldn't normally see. It's a time when everything seems to pass more slowly. The scenes are in slow motion, waking me up to what is easy to miss while revealing an intimacy I long for. Running through a town or city helps me move beyond a sense of familiarity to one of belonging. When I run, I get to know the streets, the way the lights shine from homes in the evening, the way children play in the yards, the feel of rain coming down. I discover streets I wouldn't normally know and witness the beauty of light as it cascades, heightening the beauty of everything it touches. I know the fragrances of things baking and of the seasons, fires, and the feel of fresh air through my body.

When I lived in Spain, the people had a way of asking whether you knew a place. They weren't asking so much whether you had physically been there but whether you had truly experienced it. Could I tell them the curves of the street, the way the cobblestones felt beneath my feet? Did I know the customs of the people, and had I seen the grandness and familiarity of their cathedral? Had I stopped for a coffee in the cafe around the corner, tasted the specialty food they were known for? Could I identify the murmuring sounds of their language and tell you what was most important to their hearts?

I think of the word *conoces* ("to know") sometimes when I run, wondering what the Lord is trying to tell me, what he desires for me to know—whether he wants me to know anything or just wants me to be there.

Running takes discipline, time out of the day. But often it's not wasted, as it can end up being the best part of my day, the time when I see something or feel something special that stays with me, settles in on me, and feels as if the pages of my heart have been read, giving me hope and fuel.

It seems God would want me to have more of those moments because he says he came that I might have life and loves me beyond anything I can imagine. I wonder whether he's often trying to gently tell me that I would have more of those meaningful moments if I sensed him consistently in the scenes around me, if I looked more at life through the eyes I have while running, really seeing what lies before me.

Kim

Think It Through

1. When have you enjoyed running the most? What have you learned about yourself and about God's creation during your runs?
2. Which areas of your life do you least enjoy and find yourself simply going through the motions or doing them only as a way to reach a goal?
3. What will help you enjoy the journey?
4. What "whatever" challenges are you facing that should be done for God's glory?

On Running

Does running reduce depression?

Running and exercise can reduce depression because exercise releases hormones in the body that help to elevate mood and increase energy. The greater total number of exercise sessions usually leads to a correlating decrease in depression. Greater lengths (months) of exercise also usually mean a greater reduction in depression. On the other hand, an excessive amount of exercise at one time can lead to elevated states of depression. Even though exercise can reduce depression, getting a depressed person to exercise can be difficult because that person may be fatigued, lack motivation, and have low self-esteem. Often their fitness levels are low.

JOURNAL

RUNNING LOG

	TIME	DISTANCE	WEATHER	NOTES
DAY 1				
DAY 2				
DAY 3				
DAY 4				
DAY 5				

ENJOY THE JOURNEY

You may be thinking, *Enjoying the journey while jogging around the neighborhood or doing a few quick miles sounds nice, but how about at twenty miles when I'm cramping and dizzy and can't see because of the sweat? How can that be enjoyable?* Good point. Enjoyment isn't exactly what comes to mind when you're struggling and the finish isn't in sight. So here's where we have to stretch the meaning of "enjoy" to include *help, sense, learn,* and *anticipate.* We shouldn't expect to feel good with the "runner's high" at every point of the journey.

We can enjoy our marathon experience, even during the most physically challenging times, by encouraging someone else who is also suffering, looking for faces in the crowd, and praying, thanking God for bringing us this far and asking for his strength to keep going. And here's another truth: Most marathon runners, when reflecting on their experience, will say they learned the most about themselves during those struggles and seemingly impossible miles, as they pushed through the pain and pushed ahead, sensing God working in their lives.

Listen to this amazing promise that relates to all of life, including our running exploits: "We know that God causes everything to work together for the good of those who love God and are called according to his purpose for them. For God knew his people in advance, and he chose them to become like his Son, so that his Son would be the first-born among many brothers and sisters" (Romans 8:28-29).

The Runner

Joseph had everything going for him. As the youngest of twelve boys, he was spoiled by his parents. He was also good-looking, well dressed, and had the gift of interpreting dreams. Unfortunately, he made the mistake of telling his older brothers about a dream in which he ruled over them. Here's how they responded: "'So you think you will be our king, do you? Do you actually think you will reign over us?' And they hated him all the more because of his dreams and the way he talked about them" (Genesis 37:8).

After a while, the brothers' resentment of Joseph pushed them to sell him to some traders as a slave; then they told their father that Joseph had been killed by a wild animal. Joseph was taken to Egypt, where he was purchased by an army captain named Potiphar. Joseph worked hard for Potiphar and became his personal attendant, but Potiphar's wife tried to seduce Joseph when her husband was away. When Joseph refused her advances, she screamed, "Rape!" and Joseph was put into prison.

Joseph was such a good prisoner that the warden put him in charge of all the other prisoners. One day he interpreted the dreams of a couple of men in jail with him who promised to put in a good word for Joseph when they were released. But they "forgot all about Joseph, never giving him another thought" (Genesis 40:23).

Eventually Joseph got a chance to interpret a dream for Pharaoh. And when Joseph did this successfully, Pharaoh was so impressed that he made Joseph a high official in Egypt. Then, through a series of circumstances involving a famine and food distribution, Joseph confronted his brothers who had come to Egypt for food. The brothers didn't recognize Joseph at first, but when they did, they were afraid, and rightfully so.

But listen to these words of Joseph to his brothers who had abused him and sold him into slavery: "Don't be afraid of me. Am I God, that I can punish you? You intended to harm me, but God intended it all for good. He brought me to this position so I could save the lives of many people. No, don't be afraid. I will continue to take care of you and your children" (Genesis 50:19-21).

Joseph had been torn from his family, sold into slavery, falsely accused, imprisoned, and forgotten. Yet he had seen how God had worked all of those events together for his good and God's glory.

The Race

The statement "God causes everything to work together for the good" isn't saying that *everything* is "good." It's also not implying that we'll immediately see the "good" and learn a lesson. Looking closer, we see that *God* is doing the work, not us.

The next phrase to note is "work together." This means that we shouldn't isolate certain events and wonder how they turned out to be good. Instead, God combines *all* the events to form something that is good. We must remember, too, that God can do *anything*. He can even take negative choices and experiences—our failures and sins—and make something positive from them. And then we have that word "good." This simply means something that is in our best interest, brings glory to God, and helps us to "become like his Son."

The Result

You *can* enjoy the journey, even the tough times, if you understand and believe that God is weaving these events, including your pain and difficulties, into a glorious tapestry. You may not see the final masterpiece until much later, but you can know that he is working and pulling together the strands of your life and making you like Christ. Because of this truth, you will be able—as Paul wrote to first-century believers who were encountering strong opposition and conflict—to "Always be joyful" and "Be thankful in all circumstances, for this is God's will for you who belong to Christ Jesus" (1 Thessalonians 5:16, 18).

My Story

"Layers of Dust"

RUNNING

Exposed humanity: frail body and angry thought,
Temporal distances fragmented by illusive ambitions
Cultivated by civilization, broken by wilderness: drought
Layers of dust, winter crust on skin and path; visions
Of shrill winds through frosted morning windows,
Heavy heat desiccating being: mouth and sinews.
Humbled pride—hide your face. Return?

RUNNING

Reveals redemption: cleansing mortality,
Freeing mind, external strength bracing perspective.
Nature unveils creation: colored leaves whisper,
Layers of dust—journey—snow-white roads lit by moon;
Lark song of morning brilliance, quiet painted dusk,
Undulating hills, deep forests, mirror lakes, noble peaks.
Humbled love—lifelong race: Return

Joshua

Think It Through

1. When have you faced a running obstacle you had to overcome or a problem you had to work through that you hated at the time, but then turned out to be good for you?
2. What makes seeing "good" in any situation so difficult?
3. What good has come from some of your struggles?
4. What will it take for you to "give thanks" in every situation?

On Running

What's the value of strength training?

Your workouts should have some type of resistance training. It not only strengthens ligaments and tendons, but it also increases your metabolism—building muscle and burning calories. In addition, you'll lower your heart rate and blood pressure during exertion. Your running will benefit because stronger ligaments and tendons will help keep you from rolling or spraining an ankle or knee.

JOURNAL

_____

_____

_____

_____

_____

_____

_____

_____

_____

_____

_____

_____

_____

_____

_____

RUNNING LOG

	TIME	DISTANCE	WEATHER	NOTES
DAY 1				
DAY 2				
DAY 3				
DAY 4				
DAY 5				

MAKE ADJUSTMENTS

Life is about making adjustments, adapting to changing conditions and circumstances. That's certainly true in sports. A baseball player has to try to hit the ball to the opposite field when the pitcher decides to pound the outside corner of the plate. A football offensive coordinator needs to adjust the game plan to take what the defense is giving. A basketball team should change the offensive set when the opposition switches from a man-to-man to a zone defense.

Serious runners know all about adjustments. At the beginning when they decided to run, they had to rearrange their schedules to make room. Then, when demands of work or family, storms, travel plans, or other factors interrupted the schedule, they adapted and ran at alternate times and places. Physical and emotional ailments also require adjustments (we've discussed this in Weeks 17 and 18). And those who have run long-distance races understand the necessity of adapting during the race because of equipment problems, weather conditions, physical needs, and so forth. Adjustments can include shedding unnecessary clothing as the temperature rises, working with other runners to take turns leading a line of drafters into the wind, stopping to apply petroleum jelly where needed, focusing on reaching small goals like the next aid station, and more. Being disciplined and determined is quite different from being dogmatic and set in one's ways—refusing to change. Wise runners see and feel the signs—they get the message—and adjust.

Although life is filled with potential adjustments, some people are so sure of themselves that they wouldn't change even if they were to receive a direct message from God, loud and clear and telling them what to do. And that's a problem. God speaks to us in many ways and primarily through his Word. But we need to be open and listen and hear him. This truth is mentioned often in Scripture. Check out these examples:

> *I listen carefully to what God the LORD is saying, for he speaks peace to his faithful people. But let them not return to their foolish ways.* (PSALM 85:8)

> *Listen to the words of the wise; apply your heart to my instruction. For it is good to keep these sayings in your heart and always ready on your lips. I am teaching you today—yes, you— so you will trust in the LORD.* (PROVERBS 22:17-19)

The Runner

In Week 18, we read the story of Elijah and his struggle with depression after his resounding victory over the prophets of Baal. Elijah began to recover when he rested and took nourishment. But here's what happened next:

> *The LORD said to him, "What are you doing here, Elijah?"*
> *Elijah replied, "I have zealously served the LORD God Almighty. But the people of Israel have broken their covenant with you, torn down your altars, and killed every one of your*

*prophets. I am the only one left, and now they are trying to
kill me, too."*

*"Go out and stand before me on the mountain," the LORD
told him. And as Elijah stood there, the LORD passed by, and a
mighty windstorm hit the mountain. It was such a terrible blast
that the rocks were torn loose, but the LORD was not in the wind.
After the wind there was an earthquake, but the LORD was not
in the earthquake. And after the earthquake there was a fire,
but the LORD was not in the fire. And after the fire there was
the sound of a gentle whisper. When Elijah heard it, he wrapped
his face in his cloak and went out and stood at the entrance of
the cave.* (1 KINGS 19:9-13)

Elijah had heard God, but God wanted him to listen *intently*—so
he spoke in a gentle whisper and told Elijah what to do, the adjustments to make (you can read about them in the rest of the chapter).

The Race

God can speak through catastrophic events (such as the "windstorm,"
"earthquake," and "fire") and often does. But usually he speaks in a
"gentle whisper." We have to be listening to hear his voice. That means
listening carefully, taking time in life's daily chaos to spend time in his
Word (as we discussed in Week 20). We don't have to stop to listen—
we can hear him as we walk in solitude or run and enjoy the journey.
The key is being ready, open, and tuned in to God's "gentle whisper."

The Result

If you're so busy that you don't think you can adjust your schedule to
spend time with God, you'll need to first adjust your priorities. Or if
you're the kind of person who finds changing course nearly impossible,
you'll need to ask God to soften your heart and will. God wants to
make adjustments; he wants to change your life.

My Story

As I was treading water in Lake Monona, waiting for the start cannon to fire to signal the start of Ironman Wisconsin, I wondered, *How did I get myself into this mess?*

Whatever the answer, I was there, just treading water, hanging on to a lifeguard's kayak, and waiting. I kept checking my new Garmin Forerunner 310XT GPS watch, making sure it was turned on, set for the swim leg of the race, and showing all zeroes. The latest in triathlon gadgetry, the Garmin would be my companion for the entire race. It would give me elapsed time, current speed, heart rate, distance traveled, average speed, bike pedal cadence, and even whether I was going uphill or down. It was designed to attach to a wristband while swimming or running, and with a quick twist of the watch it detached from the wristband and snapped onto a bike handlebar mount to accommodate easy viewing while riding. I had trained for a year with the Garmin and all of its electronic feedback. I was addicted to the data.

The cannon blast broke the tension, and I pushed the watch's start button, plunged my face into the water, and began to stroke. After a few hundred meters I settled into a steady pace and tried to focus on swimming straight. At the end of the first loop of the two-loop swim, I took a moment to check my watch and see how I was doing. But all I saw was a wristband—no watch face. My Garmin and all of its invaluable data was lying somewhere on the bottom of the lake—the victim of the chaotic swim start.

I felt lost, defeated, and overwhelmed. How could I pace myself on the bike without knowing how fast I was riding, how hard I was working? I would have no idea how much time had elapsed, whether I was on my projected pace, or simply how much farther I had to go. At one point, I thought I had no option but to quit at the end of the swim. It just wouldn't be possible to make it through such a challenging day without my data.

Fortunately I had another 1.2 miles to swim, to think, and to calm down. First, I had trained too long and too hard to give up so early in the race. Second, maybe I could figure out something else. Maybe I would see my daughter and borrow her sport watch. If that didn't work, maybe I could just do the whole race by feel. I mean, humans have endured a lot over the past few thousand years, and almost all of it was accomplished without a wrist-mounted GPS computer. Maybe I could tell time by judging the sun's position over the horizon!

I finally finished the swim and realized my plan of finding my daughter was ridiculous. With thousands of people cheering on family and friends at the swim exit, the chance of seeing her was minuscule. Volunteers helped me remove my wetsuit and guided me toward the bike transition.

In the transition area, another set of volunteers brought my bike gear bag—helmet, shoes, and sunglasses— and asked what else they could get for me. I noticed the sport watch on one guy's wrist and told him he could loan me his watch! I gave him my sob story, told him to put his address in my transition bag, and promised to return it to him after the race. He didn't hesitate a moment. He just took it off, tossed it to me, and wished me good luck on the rest of the race. Most important, he said, "Have fun!"

That comment recalibrated my perspective on the spot. *Oh yeah, that is why I am doing this, isn't it?*

The watch helped a little bit during the day, but most of the time on the bike I was too distracted to handle much mental math—especially because the mile markers were every fourteen miles or so. It was more helpful on the run as I could keep up with one-mile splits a little easier. Mostly I just biked and ran (and walked) as I felt I could handle it.

A little less than fourteen hours after hitting the start button on the long-lost Garmin, I found myself crossing the finish line of a long race and a long day. It was glorious. The euphoria I felt, like the anxiety at the start of the race, is also difficult to describe. I can't imagine missing out on the great sense of accomplishment that came with completing such a big challenge. To think that I had almost given up because of a bump in the road. Keeping things in their proper perspective is often tough to do, but it's so important if we are to make wise choices. I appreciated the loan of the watch, but the little phrase that refocused my thinking was invaluable.

David

P.S. My guardian angel did get his watch back, along with a gift certificate to his local triathlon shop. Also, the good folks at Garmin replaced my watch for no charge!

Think It Through

1. What big adjustments did you have to make when you began running? What adjustments have you made during a race?
2. Looking back to the time when you trusted Christ as Savior, how has your life changed because of your faith?
3. What makes hearing God's "gentle whisper" so difficult for you?
4. What can you do to be a better listener to God and to be open to what he wants you to do?

On Running

How does training help me metabolically (burning calories)?

Training increases the capacity and efficiency of metabolic systems. We can train our bodies to burn more fat during exercise. As exercise intensity increases, carbohydrates become the main energy source; whereas fat supplies more energy at lower activity levels. With training, these energy sources shift, so the need for carbohydrates as the main energy source decreases as more fat is burned. Thus, the body learns how to fuel itself and burn calories more efficiently.

JOURNAL

_____

_____

_____

_____

_____

RUNNING LOG

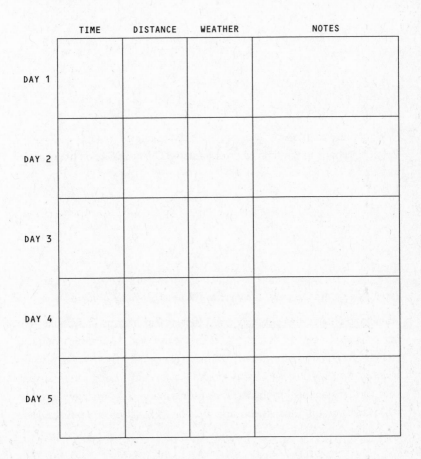

	TIME	DISTANCE	WEATHER	NOTES
DAY 1				
DAY 2				
DAY 3				
DAY 4				
DAY 5				

MAKE ADJUSTMENTS

Here's a great Bible passage for runners: "I will teach you wisdom's ways and lead you in straight paths. When you walk, you won't be held back; when you run, you won't stumble" (Proverbs 4:11-12).

The context is a father talking to his child and exhorting the child to heed his advice. The child will be wise to listen carefully and then to follow through.

We've already discussed the importance of getting good advice for running and for living (way back in Weeks 7 and 8). In running, friends who are experienced runners, coaches, running magazines, running store clerks, and other resources (including the "On Running" tips in these devotionals) can help us make important adjustments in training and more. And we have numerous Bible study tools and other resources to guide us in our spiritual races.

Last week we highlighted the importance of listening, especially to God, and hearing the adjustments he wants us to make in how we live. But if we are serious about having "straight paths" and running without stumbling, we need to take the next step—actually taking the advice and *doing it*, applying what we have heard.

The Runner

Little Megan loved watching the Olympics, especially the runners. She told her mom, "I'm going to be in the Olympics someday, probably the marathon." She would flip through magazines in the doctor's office to find pictures of people running and point them out to her parents.

As Megan grew older, she searched the Internet for running stories, especially the ones in which someone came from behind to win. She also read everything she could online about the sport. Soon she knew the history of the Olympics and could tell anyone who asked about how the marathon began and just about all the great Olympic champions, men and women. Eventually Megan subscribed to a running magazine and became an expert on everything related to running long distances: training schedules, nutrition, dealing with injuries, equipment—everything. Megan never lost her interest in all things running. Later, as an adult, she joined an online running chat room where men and women shared their running stories about the great feeling they had at setting a personal record or finishing a grueling race.

One fresh spring day, sitting in her office high above the city, Megan looked down at the running path along the lake and saw joggers making their way along the shore, avoiding walkers and cyclists. Turning from the window, she picked up the small statue of a runner she used for a paperweight and fingered it thoughtfully. *I wonder*, she mused, *if I'll ever go running.*

The Race

That story seems far-fetched, and you're probably thinking of a bunch of reasons why it would never happen. That would be like a pilot never flying, a hunter never hunting, or a singer never singing. Unfortunately, however, it's close to how some people live the Christian life. They know all about God, the Bible, and the finer points of their denomination's theology, but they don't actually *do* any of it. What they know about God and how he wants them to live doesn't affect them at all.

James has powerful advice for people like that who hear God but never follow through and make the necessary adjustments in how they live:

> *Don't just listen to God's word. You must do what it says.*
> *Otherwise, you are only fooling yourselves. For if you listen to the*
> *word and don't obey, it is like glancing at your face in a mirror.*
> *You see yourself, walk away, and forget what you look like. But*
> *if you look carefully into the perfect law that sets you free, and if*
> *you do what it says and don't forget what you heard, then God*
> *will bless you for doing it.* (JAMES 1:22-25)

The person who looks in a mirror and sees dirt on the face, disheveled hair, and a piece of spinach between the front teeth and who walks away and does nothing, thinking, *I'm looking good!* is self-deceived. People who are serious about their faith, about following Christ, will do what they know God is telling them—they will make the adjustments God wants them to make.

The Result

If you were running in a marathon and a spectator friend alongside you warned, "Watch out for the banana peels on the ground," you'd be alert and watch your step. If a veteran runner told you about shoes that could compensate for your pronation problem, you'd listen and follow that expert's advice. If at mile fourteen (out of 26.2) you felt overheated because the clouds had left, you'd remove the outer layer that you had donned for warmth. In each case, you'd hear and sense what you should do, *and then you'd do it.*

Run your race of faith the same way, listening for God's voice, hearing him, and doing what he says.

My Story

Mitch welcomed me back into the store. I hadn't seen him for almost six months, the last time I had bought a pair of running shoes. He asked me about the races I had recently run and wanted an update on how those shoes had worked out for me. We became reacquainted friends as I browsed around the local running store, which adjoined the local bike shop.

The first time I met Mitch, I came in with a dream, a big, crazy dream that made my friends and family chuckle when I told them. I planned to run a marathon. Me, just an average runner accustomed to chasing away geese while dodging their droppings all over the sidewalk on frosty mornings around the pond.

After determining to run that first marathon, I knew a good pair of shoes topped the list of things I needed. In one of my many running magazines, I remembered reading a suggestion about taking old shoes into a running store to have an expert analyze the wear patterns. Somehow this would reveal the way feet hit the pavement and where extra support is needed. Very skeptical about how much dirty soles could tell anyone, I carried a bag with my sweaty, worn-out old shoes when I first met Mitch.

True to the words of the magazine writers, he studied the sole of my shoe and declared that I suffered from overpronation. Not only did he look at my old shoes, but he also wanted to watch the way I ran in new shoes. I quickly realized his expertise in proper running-shoe fit, and my skepticism slid away under the racks of COOLMAX shirts and shorts.

The shoes he suggested to correct my tendency to overpronate and better stabilize my ankles felt like miracles on my feet. I ran for miles and miles in those shoes. On a sunny October morning, the laces securely held the time chip and led me across the finish line of my first marathon.

My running equipment did not fail me, and I vowed to return to Mitch every six months for replacement shoes.

Angie

Think It Through

1. What's more difficult in running—getting good advice or following it? Why?
2. How about in the Christian life?
3. What adjustments in how you live do you know God wants you to make?
4. What's keeping you from making them?

On Running

What should I do if someone is overheating (hyperthermia)?

Hyperthermia comes in three levels. The least concerning is heat cramps, usually caused by not being used to the heat and losing too many electrolytes. The electrolytes can be replaced with a simple sports drink. The next level is heat exhaustion. The person becomes dizzy and fatigued with a rapid pulse, and he or she probably will faint. This person needs to get to a cooler place quickly and be given lots of water. Finally, the third level, and the one of greatest concern, is heat stroke. This is when the body has stopped sweating and the skin is quite dry. The person is extremely dehydrated, with a body temperature of about 104 degrees Fahrenheit. This person should be covered in ice or put in an ice bath *immediately*.

JOURNAL

_____

_____

_____

_____

_____

_____

_____

RUNNING LOG

	TIME	DISTANCE	WEATHER	NOTES
DAY 1				
DAY 2				
DAY 3				
DAY 4				
DAY 5				

BREATHE DEEP

At almost any time during a race, we may begin to panic, thinking we'll never make it, and entertain thoughts about quitting. The miles to the finish may seem insurmountable . . . or we feel terrible . . . or we may have stumbled and fallen . . . or we've lost track of a running partner . . . or we've encountered a problem . . . or some combination of those factors. At those times, we need to take a breath, refocus, and keep going. Seriously, taking deep breaths is the perfect antidote for anxiety (and will give us more oxygen).

When worry moves beyond concern to anxiety, the next step can be panic and desperation, especially during the tough times of a long-distance run/race . . . and in life. Yet God, through Paul, tells us, "Always be full of joy in the Lord. I say it again—rejoice!" (Philippians 4:4).

Seriously, "always"? How is that possible? we might think.

So Paul tells us:

Don't worry about anything; instead, pray about everything. Tell God what you need, and thank him for all he has done. Then you will experience God's peace, which exceeds anything we can

understand. His peace will guard your hearts and minds as you
live in Christ Jesus.

And now, dear brothers and sisters, one final thing. Fix
your thoughts on what is true, and honorable, and right, and
pure, and lovely, and admirable. Think about things that are
excellent and worthy of praise. Keep putting into practice all
you learned and received from me—everything you heard from
me and saw me doing. Then the God of peace will be with you.
(PHILIPPIANS 4:6-9)

The Runner

This had not been one of Chase's better days at work—boring meetings, conflicts, and interpersonal stress seemed to fill every moment
. . . along with a call from his wife, Jill, with news that the credit card
company still hadn't corrected their mistake. He couldn't wait to leave
the office behind and get home.

"I don't believe it," Chase muttered as he walked from the building
to his car. "Snowing again." He opened the back door, threw in his
briefcase and pulled out the scraper, and began brushing snow from his
windows and mirrors, slipping and banging his bad knee against the
front bumper in the process. The ride home was excruciatingly slow as
Chase tried to avoid heavy traffic and icy patches, and the radio seemed
to have only bad news about the dismal economy.

About half an hour into his commute, his cell phone rang—a call
from a valued customer with a strong complaint. Chase did his best to
soothe the customer's feelings and solve the problem, but he wasn't too
successful. After he hung up and while trying to replace the phone, it
slipped from his hand and under the seat.

As he was about to pass the neighborhood drug store, Chase suddenly remembered that he had promised to pick up Jill's prescription,
so he pulled into the drive-thru lane . . . and waited and waited, burning gas. "What's wrong with these people!" he almost shouted. Jill

had been struggling with migraines, and they hoped this medication would help.

Suddenly his cell rang, so he undid his seatbelt and struggled to reach the phone, just out of his easy grasp under the seat. As he grabbed the ringing phone, Chase heard the sound of fabric ripping—his coat had caught and torn as he had lunged for the phone. He missed the call, but a voice mail message from *his* doctor's office said they needed to talk with him about the results of his recent blood test and something about cholesterol that he couldn't quite hear.

What's next? thought Chase as he finally pulled up to the drive-thru window. He went to pay for the prescription with his credit card, but it slipped into the dirty slush. So he struggled out, found the card, and made the transaction, spattering his newly cleaned pants in the process.

When Chase arrived home—too late to exercise and just in time for dinner—he discovered that the dog had peed on the carpet and the garbage disposal wasn't working. To top off the day, that evening as he tried to unwind, Chase watched his favorite pro basketball team stink up the court. By the time Chase slipped under the covers, he felt frustrated and angry. "Everything in my life is so screwed up!" he mumbled as he tried to fall asleep. But at 1:00 a.m. he was still tossing and turning.

The Race

Chase was having a miserable afternoon and evening, with nothing going right. At every irritation and setback, his stress and anxiety levels rose. Compared to many people, however, Chase's struggles were pretty insignificant. But small or large, irritations, conflicts, failures, and problems can affect us emotionally and spiritually and pull us down.

Not only can anxiety bring discouragement and thoughts about quitting, it can also sap our strength. In a race or in life, excessive worry leads to shortness of breath and muscle tightness and can bring on other physical problems. We feel stress and anxiety when we focus on all the negatives of our present condition, forgetting about the positive and good and about our ultimate goal.

If anyone had reason to give up, it was Job. He had lost his kids, his farm, and his health. His wife told him to "curse God and die" (Job 2:9), and his friends suggested that he had brought this calamity on himself through some secret sin. Job didn't have any answers, nor did he know what his next step should be, but he declared this about God: "Though he slay me, yet will I hope in him" (Job 13:15, NIV). Now that's an example of focus and trust!

The Result

Hopefully you won't have to endure troubles and trials as painful as Job's. But if *he* can endure, so can you. During tough times—all of them, even the daily irritations of coworkers, weather, traffic, pets, and appliances—breathe deeply from God's love. This involves remembering who he is, praying and focusing your thoughts on him, and thanking him for everything he has given you, all that is "true, and honorable, and right, and pure, and lovely, and admirable" (especially your salvation). That practice won't remove the difficulties, problems, and pain, but it will remove the anxiety and restore your strength for the journey.

My Story

Waking up early in the morning may not be everyone's cup of tea (or coffee). To be honest, it's not always mine! After I've snoozed the alarm three, four—okay, maybe five—times, I finally roll out of bed. I'm already thinking about what I need to accomplish, what I didn't finish yesterday, and fast-approaching deadlines. The weight of these thoughts makes my bed almost irresistible; yet I walk past it, down the stairs to where my shoes await. As I sit to tie my running shoes,

I sense a twinge of excitement beginning to build. When I open the door, step out into the fresh morning air, and stretch, the thoughts that earlier weighed me down seem left behind. It's just me, God, and the pavement. I begin to run, and every breath rejuvenates as I press on. Hearing the rhythm of my feet and the steadiness of my breath renews my energy. The sun paints the sky, and as the rays reach the trees, the earth seems to catch fire from the beams. Creation begins to sing, and the branches seem to reach even higher toward the heavens in praise to the Creator.

The still morning comes alive with color and joyful song, and I think, "Always be full of joy in the Lord. I say it again—rejoice! . . . Don't worry about anything; instead, pray about everything" (Philippians 4:4, 6). Rejoicing in the Lord while giving him all my anxious thoughts is not always easy. But when it is just me, God, and the pavement, I can lay my burdens at his feet, share my fears and concerns, rejoice in the victories, and enjoy his creation. This is a time not only for exercising or training but also for being one with my Creator.

As I turn the last corner and run up that last hill, though tired, I am rejuvenated. Now I can face those thoughts and concerns I left at the door, knowing I have laid them at the King's feet. "Fix your thoughts on what is true, and honorable, and right, and pure, and lovely, and admirable. Think about things that are excellent and worthy of praise" (Philippians 4:8).

When I choose to approach my day knowing the King of kings and Lord of lords will be my strength, I can live with expectations and deadlines, knowing I can daily come to him. Pondering on what is good, giving the worry over to the Lord, allows me to move through my tasks with the same vigor I feel when running, with a steadiness of mind and a confidence of spirit.

Amy

Think It Through

1. When has something during a run caused you to feel stressed or anxious? How about during a race? How did you overcome and keep running?
2. What relatively minor irritations and frustrations have stolen your joy? What major issues have sapped your strength?
3. When are you most susceptible to negative feelings about life and the future?
4. What about God and his gifts can you be thankful for? What can you do to take your eyes off your circumstances and struggles and focus on Christ?

On Running

What is positive reinforcement?

Positive reinforcement is when specific behavior is rewarded. A dog might get a treat for doing a trick. A child is rewarded with watching TV when homework is done. A runner gets a medal for finishing a marathon. These rewards help motivate a person to do what is right and to improve. There are two types of positive reinforcement rewards. Extrinsic rewards come from external sources, outside the individual, like the examples stated above. Intrinsic rewards come from within the individual, such as pride in achievement and feeling competent.

JOURNAL

RUNNING LOG

	TIME	DISTANCE	WEATHER	NOTES
DAY 1				
DAY 2				
DAY 3				
DAY 4				
DAY 5				

BREATHE DEEP

Runners often talk about getting their "second wind," newfound strength just when they feel almost too exhausted to continue. Instead of slowing dramatically or quitting, these runners continue to run at a strong pace and often exceed their expectations. Some scientists believe this phenomenon occurs when the runner's body finds enough oxygen to counteract the buildup of lactic acid in the muscles. Others think the second-wind experience is a result of endorphin production, like the "runner's high." But many believe that the feeling is psychological, an attitude adjustment and a surge of confidence caused by knowing they have passed their supposed limitations and by hearing strong encouragement from spectators and other runners. Whatever the reason, we often need a second wind in running and in life, a new, deep breath of confidence and energy.

In the first century, followers of Christ weren't very numerous or popular. Constantly persecuted and hounded by religious and secular authorities, they feared for their lives. Eventually, thousands of believers perished under cruel Roman emperors. But they remained faithful to Christ to the end because they knew the truth. Paul wrote:

That is why we never give up. Though our bodies are dying, our spirits are being renewed every day. For our present troubles are small and won't last very long. Yet they produce for us a glory that vastly outweighs them and will last forever! So we don't look at the troubles we can see now; rather, we fix our gaze on things that cannot be seen. For the things we see now will soon be gone, but the things we cannot see will last forever. (2 CORINTHIANS 4:16-18)

In some respects, those verses could have been written to a pain-riddled and exhausted marathon runner. But they also apply to anyone struggling for breath in life's marathon. Paul's advice: "Our present troubles are small and won't last very long. . . . So we don't look at the troubles we can see now; rather, we fix our gaze on things that cannot be seen." And with this change of focus and attitude comes the second wind.

The Runner

This was baby Lindsey's world—the crib, the room, the rest of the house, her mother's and father's arms. For her, nothing existed beyond all that.

Young Travis knew what the world was like; after all, he had been around the block a time or two (literally, on his tricycle). And he had been driven all over town by Mom, Dad, and big brother Tom. He also knew his way around his grandparents' homes and church. Beyond that twenty-mile radius, things got a little fuzzy, however. He thinks he remembers a long trip somewhere, but he's not sure.

Alayna has traveled quite a bit for a teenager: vacation trips with the family to the Grand Canyon out west and to the Florida Keys in the southeast. And she's studied geography in school and watched people travel the world in numerous TV shows. That's her dream, to visit those exotic locales.

Evelyn and Craig have seen and experienced much in their seventy years on the earth and nearly fifty years together. Their view of life and love has grown through those years, having lived what they had vowed at the altar: for better or worse, for richer or poorer, and in sickness and health—all of it. And they've had marvelous adventures together—ocean cruises and other trips to Asia, Europe, and Australia.

The apostle Paul hadn't traveled across the ocean and wouldn't live to be seventy. But his perspective had expanded well beyond the confines of mortal life and planet Earth. So as he sat in a Roman prison awaiting execution, he could write, "The Lord will deliver me from every evil attack and will bring me safely into his heavenly Kingdom. All glory to God forever and ever! Amen" (2 Timothy 4:18).

The Race

Interesting how one's perspective can change, and what a difference it makes!

We've been using the words "breath" and "wind." Interestingly, the Bible uses "breath" and "wind" to describe the work of the Holy Spirit (see John 20:22 and Acts 2:2). Also, the Greek word for "spirit" is *pneuma*, which means "wind." All those who have trusted in Christ as Savior have the Holy Spirit living in them, giving them strength and guidance for living and power to change. Relying fully on the Holy Spirit is, then, to focus on God, breathe deeply of him, and get our second wind. As Paul reminds us, "Though our bodies are dying, our spirits are being renewed every day." We don't have to give in and give up; with renewed attitude, focus, and strength, we can press on to the finish.

The Result

Paul's encouraging words to the Corinthians also point to the profound truth that no matter how much we work out, eat well, and avoid dangerous situations, our bodies still are "dying." Yet the "glory" to come "will last forever!" This knowledge helped Paul endure and finish strong. The way to change our attitudes is to change our perspectives, seeing our lives from God's point of view. Our current struggles won't last long in light of eternity, when we will forever run with our Savior.

Look ahead to the finish and look beyond to glory. Change your attitude and focus, breathe deeply of God's Spirit, and get your second wind.

My Story

Running in Hong Kong is an *all in* activity. The humid air almost drips with the pungent energy of Hong Kong's Kowloon neighborhood. It's hard to take an "easy" run in these conditions.

I was staging for my travels into China, where I would be teaching English at a university in Xi'an. The foundation arranging this venture boarded us in Kowloon for a few weeks to prepare us for our travels back in time.

Having never been in Asia before, I was fascinated from the moment I stepped off the plane into the thick night. I found Kowloon close to downtown, the Star Ferries, and the rail line that would whisk me into China with the same ease one boards the 'L' in Chicago. We were also close to the airport, or at least the landing pattern for it. Back then, the airport was one runway built out into the harbor directly off Kowloon City. It has since been moved. But that June, the massive underbellies of a continuous stream of 747s slid over the top of Lion Rock and plummeted to a get-it-right-the-first-time landing.

This all proved too intoxicating to resist. Lion Rock is a deserted, overgrown ridge, rising above the masses to the west. A visual destination is always a good run motivator. I had to explore.

I was up with the roosters at 5 a.m. Once onto deserted Waterloo Road, I gave a quick check of my laces, hit the watch, and off I went.

The first thing I noticed was that I was immediately

climbing. The base of Lion Rock spills down for quite a
few kilometers, and any hope of a flat warm-up was quickly
lost. "Warm-up" in general was a bit of a misnomer. The
morning air was already in the upper eighties.

Heading west on the empty streets, I soon passed the
neon of the "Romance Hotels," with patrons' expensive cars
hidden away in private parking stalls.

As I climbed out of the neighborhood, the houses gave
way to the large Beacon Hill School yard and my first view
of the shanty villages above.

The path took me higher, right through the center of
the shanty villages—literally, tin shacks crammed with
thousands of residents waiting for openings in one of the
hundreds of high-rises that define the Hong Kong skyline.
These days those shanty villages are gone, replaced with
two dozen more high-rise apartment buildings.

Crossing Lung Cheung Road, I joined a footpath
that continued toward the base of Lion Rock and into
increasingly thicker vegetation. *Still climbing. Heart
rate up. A stride not unlike stadium workouts back home,
but in a setting a world apart. Feeling very alive.*

Then the path ended. My pace slowed. My cadence and
heart rate did not. I searched for a route by taking the
next step, then the next. My hands were now involved as I
wrestled with bushes and tree trunks for balance. My route
was almost vertical now and the vegetation thick enough
that I couldn't always see where I was planting my feet.

Eventually the domed radar antenna that crowns the top
of Lion Rock came into view, the vegetation dropped away,
and as I turned around, I was rewarded with a magnificent
view of the sunrise over the harbor, the light dancing
off the South China Sea, its expanse littered with ships
awaiting their turn in port.

I learned long ago that cameras don't work in moments
like this. With my heart rate settling after a good
effort, endorphins flowing, sweat rolling, and the feeling
of being alive that only a run can produce, all the

photographs in the world wouldn't come close. I noticed a number of cuts on my arms and legs, and a subtle amount of blood mixing with the sweat. Lion Rock had autographed me. A badge of honor. That was my photograph.

After taking in the city in all its dimensions, I walked over to the radar installation, where I discovered a very narrow, very tidy road winding down the back side of Lion Rock. I laughed, but not with regret. I hit the watch, and off I went.

Making my way back into the heart of Kowloon, I passed a white tour bus getting an early start at seeing the sights. Faces appeared in rank order, imprisoned behind the tinted glass. Air-conditioned. Sterile.

I felt sorry for those folks. They would never know Hong Kong the way I did. I had run in Hong Kong. I had bled in Hong Kong. I had it under my skin.

Todd

Think It Through

1. When have you gotten a second wind in a long run or a long-distance race? How did you feel? What do you think was the cause?
2. How has your perspective changed as you have grown older, gained knowledge, and experienced life's ups and downs?
3. How do you know that your future in heaven with Christ is secure?
4. In what ways does that knowledge give you hope right now, especially during trying circumstances?

On Running

What is overtraining?

Overtraining is a condition in which an athlete's adaptive mechanisms (increased oxygen uptake, increased muscle strength, and improved lactic threshold) are stressed to the point of failure. Feeling "burned out," the body failing to heal itself, and further training that doesn't improve performance (possibly even causing a drop in performance) are all signs of overtraining. Some symptoms include poor practices, poor performance, weight loss, joint and muscle pain without injury, nausea, a head cold/stuffy nose, depression, irritability, insomnia, and anxiety.

You can avoid overtraining by designing a training program with variety and that alternates hard and easy days (you may need more than twenty-four hours for recovery). If you are feeling overtrained, rest—start with two days of rest. Then, if you still have symptoms, increase to five days. And eat well. A high-carbohydrate diet aids in recovery.

JOURNAL

_____

_____

_____

_____

_____

_____

_____

_____

_____

_____

_____

_____

_____

_____

_____

_____

RUNNING LOG

	TIME	DISTANCE	WEATHER	NOTES
DAY 1				
DAY 2				
DAY 3				
DAY 4				
DAY 5				

BE PATIENT

One of the first lessons learned by long-distance runners is patience. That's not the case for sprinters, who start as fast as possible and measure each race in seconds. When the run is more than a mile, successful competitors understand that the race is won at the *end*, not the beginning, so they pace themselves in order to have energy and stamina when they need them. Many marathons—such as New York, Boston, and Chicago—draw tens of thousands of runners, and all those behind the elite competitors at the front learn another lesson in patience as they weave around and through other runners the whole way, patiently working their way forward. Runners also learn patience by enduring a variety of aches, pains, and inconveniences such as poor weather conditions. And this may seem obvious, but they know they can't finish a marathon unless they run 26.2 miles—not easy for anyone.

Pain is part of the process; but without the pain, runners won't gain the prize and the joy of competing well and finishing strong. Runners also know that they grow stronger by running through the hard times of a race.

This is true of life in general, not just in running. It's a truth emphasized in a familiar Bible passage:

Dear brothers and sisters, when troubles come your way, consider it an opportunity for great joy. For you know that when your faith is tested, your endurance has a chance to grow. So let it grow, for when your endurance is fully developed, you will be perfect and complete, needing nothing. (JAMES 1:2-4)

Now there's a challenge: "Consider [your troubles] an opportunity for great joy." That will take patience indeed.

The Runner

Heather jogged along the path that wound through her town, just a light run to give her a chance to take a much-needed break to gather her thoughts.

"I need a decision by tomorrow," her boss had said. "This is a great opportunity that may never come again, and I think you'd be foolish not to take it."

The offered promotion sounded so inviting—more responsibility, increased salary, opportunities to travel. But Heather wasn't comfortable with the values of the company and actually had been thinking of quitting. "What should I do, Lord?" she whispered as she ran. "How can I pass this up?"

And then, almost in time with her strides, she sensed God whispering back, "Patience . . . trust me . . . patience . . . trust me."

Patience had never been Heather's strong suit. As a baby, her favorite expression had been "Now!" And as a child, she would hunt for her Christmas presents around the house—she couldn't wait until December 25. But she could remember her father saying, "Be patient, Heather, and trust me. You'll love Christmas!" She also remembered family vacation trips when she would continually ask, almost plead, "Are we there yet? How much longer?" and Mom would tell her to be patient, that the destination would be worth the trip. Another great test of patience had been the braces on her teeth—right at thirteen when she was beginning to be concerned about how she looked. "You'll have to be patient," Aunt Barb had told her. "You'll only have them a couple of years, but your new smile will be worth it."

Wait . . . patience . . . trust! Those three words seemed to always go together. And Heather had to admit, her dad, mom, and aunt had been right. The thought stopped her on the path, and tears formed as she prayed, "Forgive me, Lord, for thinking I know best and for being so impatient. Help me to trust you."

And Heather made her decision.

The Race

When we receive a promise, we can patiently wait for it to be ful-filled *if* we trust the person making the promise. The Bible high-lights many promises of God to us, offering us hope. In places like the passage in James, it's as if God is saying, "Hang in there. Trust me. Your troubles are building you up, and soon everything will be all right—you'll see." And if we pass this test of faith and learn this lesson of growing endurance, we'll be ready for anything and experience "great joy."

The Result

As you consider how patient you are, remember that it's a matter of trust. And hear this amazing promise that should motivate you in every race:

> *Those who trust in the LORD will find new strength. They will soar high on wings like eagles. They will run and not grow weary. They will walk and not faint.* (ISAIAH 40:31)

My Story

"And why do you run?" is a question I get from people who think I'm slightly odd at best and deranged at worst. Depending on my mood, I might answer, "Because I hope I can."

There is truth to my answer, especially because I began running long distances in my midforties and entered my first marathon, Chicago 2009, in my early fifties. Over the next decade I want to run my four "biggies": New York, San Diego, Houston, and finally (Lord willing) qualify for the Boston.

I ran my first 5K in 1973 as a freshman on the cross-country team. Although at most practices I ran a 10:30-mile pace, placing me among the last third of my teammates, for that event I had pictured myself winning the race ahead of even seniors who could run a 6:30-mile pace.

When the gun sounded, I flew ahead of everyone as if I had wings on my heels, putting a fifty-yard distance between me and the others. I glanced back at the shrinking runners behind me and thought, *This isn't so hard.*

Then at the quarter-mile turn, something awful happened: My side began aching, my breathing became heavy, and my legs slowed to a trot. Then my pride took a serious (though necessary) blow as all fifty runners breezed past me. By the mile-one marker, I could not run another step. I walked ever so slowly and sheepishly back to the start, never to finish my first cross-country race. I did, however, complete that one and only season of cross-country, usually running in the back third of the pack.

Fast-forward thirty-three years to a cold October Saturday morning in Grant Park, where I and more than forty thousand other runners lined up to run the Chicago Marathon. This time I had no visions of a great finish and had strategically placed myself in the middle of the pack with the ten-minute-mile pacesetters.

After the national anthem and the raining down of discarded sweat pants and shirts, I began to finish what I started back at my first cross-country race. And when I hit the wall this time (about mile eighteen), I kept running. From then on, though, I must admit that after each water station I found the stiffness and ache in both knees harder to ignore as I returned to my running.

At mile twenty-five, a runner just to my left collapsed suddenly to the asphalt from severe cramping in both of his calves. *Do I keep going and finish or stop and help?* I wondered. I stopped, bent down, and helped him sit up while a runner from Atlanta with whom I had been running the last three miles motioned for race personnel. For the moment, I forgot that I was only one short mile from the finish. Under the capable hands of race officials, the exhausted man slowly got up and limped off to the side of Michigan Avenue.

My running partner and I looked at each other, both feeling our own cramping, and looked north toward the finish. In those first few steps, the ache screamed from every muscle in my legs and back, "Why are you running?"

I did not answer myself. Instead, with every step, the pain lessened and my pace increased as I could hear the crowd at the finish line with the announcer's voice from tower-high speakers cheering the runners on to the finish.

Then it happened: After four hours, thirty-two minutes, I crossed the finish line. I had run the Chicago Marathon.

As special as finishing my first marathon was, I anticipate an even greater finish in "the race God has set before" me. In this one, together with all Christians, we keep "our eyes on Jesus, the champion who initiates and perfects our faith" (Hebrews 12:1-2). Crossing that finish line will be glorious!

Michael

Think It Through

1. What examples of impatience can you remember from your childhood? What event(s) did you find it most difficult to wait for?
2. At what times have you had to be patient for something that you discovered was definitely worth the wait?
3. Besides running, what else has taught you to be patient? Why is trusting God so difficult during tough times?
4. What do you sense God telling you to patiently wait for?

On Running

Why is self-confidence so important for runners?

Self-confidence is the belief that you can successfully perform a desired behavior. This attitude has a number of benefits. Your confidence helps arouse positive emotions, causing you to react more positively to adversity. Confidence improves concentration, increases effort (be sure to set challenging goals), and intimidates the opponent. Most important, you are more relaxed and have more fun!

JOURNAL

_____

_____

_____

_____

_____

_____

_____

_____

RUNNING LOG

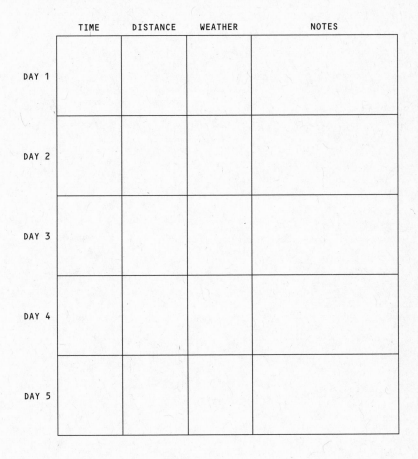

	TIME	DISTANCE	WEATHER	NOTES
DAY 1				
DAY 2				
DAY 3				
DAY 4				
DAY 5				

BE PATIENT

You may have heard these familiar clichés concerning patience: "Good things come to those who wait," "Patience is a virtue," and "Hurry up and wait." Another one that occurs in Scripture is the phrase "patient endurance," implying that patience involves putting up with something unpleasant for a long time—that's why it has been translated "long-suffering." Those sitting in a boring lecture or meeting understand a bit of this idea. Those who have had to endure complicated dental work understand it too. Runners know the feeling of "suffering" for a "long" time, usually beginning in the serious stage of a race and continuing until the finish. Runners need patience during those long miles for sure!

In the Bible, patience is often cited in the context of experiencing hardships or enduring suffering for Christ (much more severe than meetings, teeth problems, and marathons) and waiting for Christ's glorious return and heavenly rewards. Here's an example:

Think back on those early days when you first learned about Christ. Remember how you remained faithful even though it meant terrible suffering. Sometimes you were exposed to public ridicule and were beaten, and sometimes you helped others who were suffering the same things. You suffered along with those who were thrown into jail, and when all you owned was taken from you, you accepted it with joy. You knew there were better things waiting for you that will last forever.

So do not throw away this confident trust in the Lord. Remember the great reward it brings you! Patient endurance is what you need now, so that you will continue to do God's will. Then you will receive all that he has promised. (HEBREWS 10:32-36)

Peter gives another powerful example, writing to people who were undergoing great persecution, including torture and death—"fiery trials." Here's his message:

Dear friends, don't be surprised at the fiery trials you are going through, as if something strange were happening to you. Instead, be very glad—for these trials make you partners with Christ in his suffering, so that you will have the wonderful joy of seeing his glory when it is revealed to all the world. (1 PETER 4:12-13)

Today, people are still suffering for Christ.

The Runner

On May 7, 2009, two members of a Colombian guerrilla group burst into the home of church leader José Rodriguez and his wife, Emilse Maria del Carmen, and shot them dead in front of two of their children, Heidy (9) and Ambar (2). When the grandparents and neighbors arrived to take care of the bodies, Heidy took her sister's hand and led her outside. Someday the girls and their brother, Juan (2 mos.), may understand that their parents were Christian martyrs—murdered because they believed in Christ. But now, all Heidy could do was whisper in Ambar's ear, "My parents now are in heaven. And we—we are under Lord Jesus."

Christians in Al-Nawahid, Egypt, were attacked on November 15, 2010, by hundreds of Muslims who rampaged through their community, firebombing houses and businesses after hearing rumors of a romantic relationship between a Christian and a Muslim. Though the rumor proved untrue, the resulting violence reflects a feud among three families vying for political control in the area, using Christians as targets in an effort to unseat the town's mayor.

Officials in Katin village (Laos) ordered six more Christian families to renounce their faith or face expulsion in early January 2011. Eleven Christian families, totaling forty-eight people, were expelled at gunpoint in January 2010. The six families now under threat had become Christians since the January expulsion. In July 2010, village leaders said they would shoot every Christian who returned to Katin.

In Somalia on November 25, 2010, seventeen-year-old Nurta Mohamed Farah, who converted to Christianity from Islam, was shot to death in an apparent "honor killing."

On November 5, 2010, a private investigation team visited four villages in Kandhamal district (India), Orissa state, the site of anti-Christian violence in 2008. Christians reported that the local administration had done little to protect them, and they suspected that officials had colluded with area Hindu nationalists. Many Christians are still ostracized and pressured to return to Hinduism. Recent incidents of persecution in states other than Orissa include Hindu extremists beating a Christian, three Christian gatherings disrupted, a Christian burial blocked, and false complaints against Christians registered with the police.

In Vietnam, two Christian evangelists, Ksor Y Du and Kpa Y Co, received harsh sentences of six and four years in prison, respectively, for "undermining national unity." Both evangelists, who are of the Ede minority, were arrested and held ten months without charges. Ksor was one of many thousands of ethnic minority people who had demonstrated in 2004 against religious oppression and illegal confiscation of their traditional lands.

(These reports of courageous believers are adapted from reports by Open Doors, www.opendoorsusa.org.)

The Race

Clearly, followers of Christ are still being persecuted for their faith. The early believers experienced *extreme* suffering, yet they could rejoice because they knew that in light of eternity, their time of suffering was short, and they knew that what awaited them after death was worth anything they might have to endure in life. That's why Paul could write, "I am glad when I suffer for you in my body, for I am participating in the sufferings of Christ that continue for his body, the church" (Colossians 1:24).

During his ministry for Christ, Paul was given thirty-nine lashes five times; three times he was beaten with rods; once he was stoned; he was slandered and chased from cities; he experienced two Roman prison terms; eventually, he was executed—all because he dared to live and speak boldly for Christ (see 2 Corinthians 11:24-27). Now that's "patient endurance"!

The Result

You probably won't be lashed thirty-nine times, beaten with rods, or stoned. But you will endure hardships because of your faith. When that happens, learn from your running experiences and the powerful examples of Peter, Paul, and the early church. Rejoice in your sufferings as you confidently and patiently press forward for Christ.

My Story

When I considered running a marathon, veteran runners encouraged me to train for the Mardi Gras Marathon. They said it would be a good one because of the size (2,000+

runners) and the straight course—we would be running across
the world's longest bridge, the Lake Pontchartrain Causeway,
which spans more than twenty-three miles. Besides, the start
would be just about three or four miles from my house in
Covington. (The race would begin two miles before the bridge
and finish about a mile after the bridge, in Metairie.)
Sounded good to me—so I trained during October, November,
and December for the race in early January.

What a disaster! When I awoke and prepared for the
race, I learned that a warm front had moved in, so we
would be running *into* the wind. And because of the
straight course, the wind would be in my face *the entire
race*—at thirty-five miles per hour. Also, I soon realized
that running over a bridge meant no spectators to cheer us
on. Except for the aid stations, we runners were on our
own. Speaking of no encouragement, we had nothing to look
at except water on the right and concrete in front and
on the left—not very inspiring. Early on, I noticed that
many were running in small lines or columns, protecting
each other from the wind by taking turns leading the pack
and drafting off each other. Unfortunately, being six foot
three, I couldn't duck behind anyone.

I was struggling when I came to the second high-rise—
hills in the causeway for boats to pass under, at mile
markers eight and sixteen. I saw runners walking up the
incline, and I thought, *I'll keep running. Then when I get
to the top, I'll see the other shore and I'll be running
downhill! That ought to inspire me and give me my second
wind.*

Instead, after exerting the last of my energy to get
to the top, I suddenly felt the full force of the wind—
it had been partially blocked by the bridge. Instead of
running downhill, because of the wind it seemed as if
I were running on flat ground. And yes, I could see the
shoreline, but it was still about *five miles* away.

A worker tried to be encouraging by saying, "Just a 10K
left," but I thought, *More than six miles? I'll never make
it.* I definitely had slammed into the wall. Small buses

passed periodically to pick up runners who had given up. I seriously considered it. But I thought of all the training I had invested—wasted. I also knew that I would be second-guessing myself about the decision for months and years to come. But mainly I kept going because I knew that my wife, Gail, and our six-year-old daughter, Kara, would be waiting for me at the finish.

I had nothing left—absolutely nothing—yet I kept going somehow. I don't remember the next few miles at all, just one foot in front of the other, running, shuffling, walking . . . moving forward until my feet hit land and through bleary eyes I saw the crowds and heard their cheers. I stumbled along and then straightened up as I turned the corner onto Veterans Highway and saw the finish . . . and gave it my all.

The next day's headlines read, "Few Survive Causeway Killer." I was one.

Dave

Think It Through

1. What's the most painful experience you've run through? What kept you going? What was your reward for finishing?
2. What has your faith in Christ cost you? What pain have you endured—or are you enduring—because you follow him?
3. What lessons has God taught you through those times of persecution? What did you (or will you) receive for enduring?
4. What lessons from Scripture will help you endure suffering for Christ in the days and years to come?

On Running

How do I build my self-confidence?

Successes build self-confidence. If you are training for a race, structure your training sessions to incorporate successes—completing a distance, running under a certain time, etc. Physical conditioning also affects a person's confidence—the better shape you are in, the better you will feel. Acting confidently will help you feel more confident—the emotion follows the act. Think confidently by focusing on the task and motivating thoughts. Avoid judgmental thoughts. Finally, the use of imagery builds self-confidence—if you see yourself engaging in something and doing it correctly, you will begin to feel more confident in that activity.

JOURNAL

RUNNING LOG

	TIME	DISTANCE	WEATHER	NOTES
DAY 1				
DAY 2				
DAY 3				
DAY 4				
DAY 5				

RECEIVE ENCOURAGEMENT

Some people act like Lone Rangers; that is, they seem to pull back from people and do everything by themselves, on their own. That can be a sign of strength, of course. These people are disciplined self-starters who don't need to be pushed, prodded, and exhorted to get moving and do the job.

Runners often run by themselves, out of necessity or by choice (up at dawn and out the door). Braving the elements and pushing through, day after day, builds character and determination. People who discipline themselves to pull on the outfit, lace up the shoes, and run no matter what are likely to be disciplined in other areas. Employers and coaches *love* having people with those qualities on their teams.

On the other hand, rugged individualism can have a dark side. Loners like this can be harmful to a team when they think their way is the only way and don't want to work with anyone else. "I'd rather do it myself, thank you very much!" is not a great attitude for a team. And those who dogmatically insist that their way is the only way may be heading blindly in the wrong direction.

No matter how strong we are individually, we need others—at least one more person—to affirm and encourage us and keep us on the right path.

Paul certainly was a strong individualist and leader. He could face angry mobs and Roman officials without fear. Even as a prisoner, he told the commanding officer what to do on their sinking ship (Acts 27:27-44). Yet Paul always had traveling companions on his lengthy mission trips—Barnabas, John Mark, Silas, Luke, and others. And he submitted himself to the leadership, counsel, and encouragement of other church leaders. Check this out:

> *Fourteen years later I went back to Jerusalem again, this time with Barnabas; and Titus came along, too. I went there because God revealed to me that I should go. While I was there I met privately with those considered to be leaders of the church and shared with them the message I had been preaching to the Gentiles. I wanted to make sure that we were in agreement, for fear that all my efforts had been wasted and I was running the race for nothing. And they supported me and did not even demand that my companion Titus be circumcised, though he was a Gentile.* (GALATIANS 2:1-3)

The Runner

Although he knew lots of runners and enjoyed talking running with many of them at work and at church, Gary ran alone. *Trying to match up with someone just isn't worth the effort,* he thought. Gary's work schedule varied, and his running schedule changed along with it, so he figured he'd have a tough time finding someone to be that flexible. He also didn't join in the weekend runs some invited him to. Gary wasn't antisocial, he simply would rather run by himself, keeping his own pace, deep in his own thoughts and enjoying nature.

Some friends mentioned running in the marathon coming up in about six months. Gary didn't say anything to them about his plans, but he decided to try it too. Up till then, his longest race had been a 10K. So he registered and carefully followed the training schedule he found online. When the race came, Gary was ready. Working his way to the start, he saw some of his friends—but carefully avoiding them, he tried to blend in with some strangers.

As the race progressed, Gary was doing well, keeping his pace and right on schedule. But he began to have breathing problems at about mile seventeen—a painful stitch in the side. He slowed and then walked and seemed to get some relief, so he began to run again. But just a few miles later, Gary hit the wall. He felt totally spent and could feel every pain—the blisters, the muscle aches, the dried sweat around his eyes, the burning lungs . . . and the stitch had returned. And he was in a stretch of the racecourse with no spectators because of the terrain. Gary walked, more like hobbled, but he kept moving.

Off to his right, he thought he heard his name. "Gary. Hey, dude, how're you doing?" Gary saw Terrance from church. Terrance looked awful and was limping along, slightly hunched over. He came up to Gary, slowed to a walk, and put his hand on Gary's shoulder. "We can do it, Gary! You're looking good. We're almost there."

Gary managed a thin smile, whispered, "Thanks," and started to run again. Thirty minutes later they crossed the finish line together.

The Race

Gary didn't think he needed anyone, but Terrance proved to be a huge encouragement. No one should try to go it alone in life. We all need help; we need people to come alongside, like Terrance, and encourage us.

Paul did. In addition to submitting himself to other church leaders, he was open to words of encouragement, especially from those who would share how Christ had changed their lives. So in anticipation of traveling to Rome to see believers in that great city, Paul wrote, "When we get together, I want to encourage you in your faith, but I also want to be encouraged by yours" (Romans 1:12).

And here's what he said to the believers in Corinth about specific individuals:

> *Be on guard. Stand firm in the faith. Be courageous. Be strong.*
> *And do everything with love.*
> *You know that Stephanas and his household were the first*
> *of the harvest of believers in Greece, and they are spending*
> *their lives in service to God's people. I urge you, dear brothers*
> *and sisters, to submit to them and others like them who*
> *serve with such devotion. I am very glad that Stephanas,*
> *Fortunatus, and Achaicus have come here. They have been*
> *providing the help you weren't here to give me. They have been*
> *a wonderful encouragement to me, as they have been to you.*
> *You must show your appreciation to all who serve so well.*
> (1 CORINTHIANS 16:13-18)

We need people to affirm, correct, encourage, and lead us.

The Result

Spending time with others and being open to them isn't always easy. As with running, you may have to adjust your pace to match theirs. But God created us to be in relationship, in community. Even Jesus surrounded himself with twelve close followers, and he sent them out two by two. Along your route, invite someone to come alongside; talk, pray, listen, and encourage each other on the way.

My Story

My wife and I trained for months to run a half marathon together—plodding every step, side by side. It was a great experience. Unfortunately, the day before the big race, my wife suffered a miscarriage and was unable to run the race. She insisted I run without her. It was a

long, hard, lonely race. But every few miles, I'd see
her standing on the sidelines cheering me on. I had a
bitter taste in my mouth as I crossed the finish line
while my best friend and running buddy had to sit on
the sidelines.

But perhaps that was a blessing in disguise. Two years
later, we trained together again. Every step, side by
side. It is so fun to run with someone and to have a
quiet voice encouraging you along the way. This year,
we finished together, hand in hand. I wouldn't trade the
experience for anything.

My advice to runners: Don't do it alone. Train with
someone. The journey is much better with a friend.

Matthew

Think It Through

1. When do you run by yourself? What do you like about running alone?
   What do you enjoy about running with someone else?
2. When has someone been a great encouragement to you by his or her
   example? When has someone, either solicited or not, encouraged you
   verbally?
3. When have you needed encouragement but were afraid to ask for it?
4. What keeps you from opening up to others? What would you like
   someone to know about you?

On Running

How will high altitude affect my training?

The biggest difference you'll notice when training at high altitudes is the
increased rate of respiration. That is, the higher you go, the less oxygen is in
the air; so you will have less oxygen in the blood. Therefore, you will breathe
more rapidly to try to get as much oxygen into your body as possible. You'll
find that you can't train at the same intensity at high altitudes as you did at
sea level.

JOURNAL

_____

_____

_____

_____

_____

RUNNING LOG

	TIME	DISTANCE	WEATHER	NOTES
DAY 1				
DAY 2				
DAY 3				
DAY 4				
DAY 5				

RECEIVE ENCOURAGEMENT

Thus far, when we've discussed the marathon experience, we've seen the start, the competitive stage, and the serious stage. The next portion of the race is the *encouragement* stage. At about twenty miles or so, runners are exhausted—feet sore and blistered, legs aching, eyes burning, and lungs bursting. But having passed the point of no return, of quitting, they know that somehow, some way, they will finish. That's when runners feel camaraderie with others who are experiencing the same struggle. Oftentimes, complete strangers, running, limping, or walking at the same pace, will decide to run together, encouraging and motivating each other to the finish.

As with the other marathon stages, this one parallels life. At some point, not always but usually in the older years, we hit the wall of adversity. Then someone comes alongside, serving, listening, affirming, counseling, and praying—and we gain strength and courage to endure. We can also be encouraged by seeing or recalling the examples of people who have successfully navigated the same troubled waters. That's what James was doing in this passage, referring to Job: "We give great honor to those who endure under suffering. For instance, you know about Job, a man of great endurance. You can see how the Lord was kind to him at the end, for the Lord is full of tenderness and mercy" (James 5:11).

Reading the stories of our brothers and sisters in Christ who have run the same path and have made it through can be a great encouragement. We've already highlighted the first few verses of Hebrews 12 a few times, but listen again to verse one:

> *Therefore, since we are surrounded by such a huge crowd of witnesses to the life of faith, let us strip off every weight that slows us down, especially the sin that so easily trips us up. And let us run with endurance the race God has set before us.*

The "huge crowd of witnesses" refers to our great heritage of faith, including all the spiritual giants mentioned in the previous chapter and so many others, right up to the present. The writer is saying that knowing that these men and women faithfully ran the race should motivate us to do the same.

The Runner

Marjorie needed to lose weight; she knew that for sure. Dieting had helped a little, but the doctor said that exercise would be best. "Why don't you try running?" he suggested.

Never having had any interest in sports, Marjorie was intimidated and fearful, but she decided to try. At first, she ran and walked a few blocks. After a couple of months, she was shedding pounds and running a mile, though it was tough. After a year or so, she added a mile . . . and then another. Then the unthinkable—a few years in, she announced to her husband, Dan, that she wanted to run a marathon . . . and she did.

So inspired by his wife's dedication, desire, and accomplishment (he knew the pain she endured in training and in the race), Dan decided to try for a marathon. Although Dan had played high school football and basketball, he had never run long distances. And at six foot four and 235 pounds, he seemed too big to make it 26.2 miles . . . but he did.

Breck couldn't believe that his buddy Dan would even try to run a marathon, much less finish. So when Dan told him about the experience and showed him the medal, Breck thought, *If Dan can do it, so can I.* His goal was to run the marathon the next year, maybe even with Dan. When Dan agreed, they trained together, pushing each other through the rough patches . . . and Breck reached his goal.

Chrissy, Breck's sister, had laughed when she first heard about his goal. *He's too lazy to do that*, she thought. So she was shocked at Breck's dedication and determination, and even more surprised that he finished and had the blisters and stories to prove it. Inspired by Breck's accomplishment, Chrissy started running and now runs every other day . . . with Marjorie. They're planning to run a marathon this year—together.

The Race

Each of those individuals was encouraged by someone else's example—someone who persevered, endured, experienced hardship and pain, and made it through. But that's running. We also find examples of friends who have fought through depression, achieved a lofty academic goal, conquered a severe illness, reinvented themselves in their careers, reared physically or developmentally disabled children, survived a failed marriage, recovered from bankruptcy, and more. These examples encourage us to keep going, despite incredible odds.

But the greatest example of suffering and endurance is our Lord himself. Return again to Hebrews 12: "Think of all the hostility he endured from sinful people; then you won't become weary and give up" (verse 3).

Paul also turned the spotlight on the Savior:

> *Though [Jesus] was God, he did not think of equality with God as something to cling to. Instead, he gave up his divine privileges;*

he took the humble position of a slave and was born as a human being. When he appeared in human form, he humbled himself in obedience to God and died a criminal's death on a cross.
(PHILIPPIANS 2:6-8)

The Result

Wherever you are in the race, be open and ready for encouragement—from others who will run with you, from the great examples of others who have run and finished the course, and most of all, from Jesus. Every temptation you've faced, every pain you've felt, and every struggle you've endured, he has too. What an example! What a Savior! And here's the best news: He's running with you.

"So encourage each other and build each other up, just as you are already doing" (1 Thessalonians 5:11).

My Story

I grew up in Zimbabwe, Africa, where every student was expected to participate in after-school activities. So I had the chance to try all sorts of sports, from cricket to swimming to track. But I excelled most in team sports like soccer, volleyball, and field hockey. My family returned to the States when I was a senior in high school, and I studied that year in a small public school in South Carolina. I was anxious to get involved in a sports program there, but they didn't offer soccer, and they sure didn't offer boys volleyball or field hockey! I didn't even attempt football or baseball. I tried out for basketball but quit before the coach could cut me from the team. The only sports that remained were golf or track. I decided to go for the latter.

I had never been a star athlete at my school in Zimbabwe, but I enjoyed running and had been jogging in the mornings for several months. Now, with some training from my coach,

I began to improve. My races were the 800 meters and the mile. I did best at the mile. For the first time in my life, I began to win some competitions, and my times were improving almost every week, going from a six-minute mile to five and a half to just above five minutes.

The day came for our first major competition: the Regional meet. That meet would decide who would go on to Upper-State and finally to State. I remember the feeling in my stomach before the start. And I remember how, just as with every other race, I scanned the track and imagined in my mind at what pace I would run each of the four grueling laps. My family was there in the stands ready to cheer me on.

The gun sounded, and the pounding of feet echoed the beating of my own heart. The first lap . . . I managed to stay with the top runners. The second lap . . . a few stragglers started falling behind. The third lap . . . going strong but wondering how long I could keep this pace. Then into the fourth and final lap . . . just one runner ahead of me. And I felt complacency, that my tired body is doing the best it can just to keep up, so why try to win now?

But then I heard a voice—no, a yell—from the stands on the far side of the track. I knew the sound well, having heard it many times before—at soccer games, cross-country events, track meets: Dad cheering for me at the top of his lungs. I knew the rest of my family was cheering too, just not as loud. And in that moment, as I rounded the corner for the last two hundred meters, I said to myself, "Well, I guess I better give them something to cheer for."

I left my halfhearted attempt behind in the dust of the track and dug down as deep as I could. I focused straight ahead and pulled hard toward the guy in front of me. As I gained on him, I could hear the cheers become louder and wilder. The rush of excitement and determination fueled my legs and allowed my body to forget its pain. Fifty meters from the finish line, my competitor lost his strength and I sprinted past, crossing the finish line in first place!

That race is forever etched in my memory, the race when the support of my family helped me abandon mediocrity and my feeling of inability and enabled me to reach for more than I thought was possible.

Mark

Think It Through

1. When you were at the stage of the race where you were tempted to become complacent, who came alongside to encourage you?
2. Who has played the role of encourager in your life?
3. What have your friends and family done to encourage you?
4. In what ways has Jesus' example given you strength and endurance?

On Running

What should I look for in a sports drink?

First, you should look at the amount of carbohydrates. The drink should have 5–10 percent carbohydrates (8 percent is ideal). More than 10 percent carbohydrates will slow down the uptake of glucose (a form of sugar for energy). Also, check the pH—if the solution is very acidic (for example, orange juice), it will slow gastric emptying and delay the body's absorption of the needed nutrients.

JOURNAL

_____

_____

_____

_____

_____

RUNNING LOG

	TIME	DISTANCE	WEATHER	NOTES
DAY 1				
DAY 2				
DAY 3				
DAY 4				
DAY 5				

GIVE ENCOURAGEMENT

Encouragement goes both ways, of course. We need people to give us a boost, to affirm and compliment us, to pray for us, and to urge us on. We also need good examples to emulate. And we need this at every point along the race and in life, but especially during those bumps, setbacks, and challenges. At the same time, we should be looking for people *we* can encourage.

In running, being an encourager can start when someone begins to consider becoming a "runner." Many runners say they entered the sport at the urging of a friend and that the two friends held each other accountable for keeping to a regular running schedule. And many runners have running partners, friends who meet at the park to run a trail or at the fitness center to run around the track or neighbors who meet up and run through the neighborhood. The runs become social events.

We've already discussed the importance of encouragement in long-distance races, especially in the later stages during physical and emotional stress. We may find that running with a loved one or friend is difficult in a race because of the differences in pace and physical needs and the press of the pack. But we still can find runners, even strangers, to come alongside and encourage us on the way.

God has a lot to say about how his people should relate to others. He expects us to care for the needy (Matthew 25:34-40), treat others as we want to be treated (Matthew 7:12), love our "neighbors" (Matthew 22:39), and serve (John 13:34-35). In addition, our acts of loving service and words of encouragement should touch all kinds of people—children, spouses, neighbors, believers, unbelievers, widows, aliens, and even enemies (can you say "competitors"?). And we should point them to the ultimate Encourager, "the source of all comfort." This passage pretty much says it all:

> *All praise to God, the Father of our Lord Jesus Christ. God is our merciful Father and the source of all comfort. He comforts us in all our troubles so that we can comfort others. When they are troubled, we will be able to give them the same comfort God has given us. For the more we suffer for Christ, the more God will shower us with his comfort through Christ. Even when we are weighed down with troubles, it is for your comfort and salvation! For when we ourselves are comforted, we will certainly comfort you. Then you can patiently endure the same things we suffer. We are confident that as you share in our sufferings, you will also share in the comfort God gives us.* (2 CORINTHIANS 1:3-7)

The Runner

> *When the church at Jerusalem heard what had happened, they sent Barnabas to Antioch. When he arrived and saw this evidence of God's blessing, he was filled with joy, and he encouraged the believers to stay true to the Lord. Barnabas was a good man, full of the Holy Spirit and strong in faith. And many people were brought to the Lord.* (ACTS 11:22-24)

Every group needs an "encourager," because everyone needs encouragement at one time or another. The value of encouragement is often missed, however, because it tends to be private rather than public. In fact, people most need encouragement when they feel most alone. A man named Joseph was such an encourager that he earned the nickname "Son of Encouragement," or Barnabas, from the Jerusalem Christians (Acts 4:36).

Barnabas was drawn to people he could encourage, and he was a great help to everyone around him. Barnabas's actions were crucial to the early church. In a way, we can thank him for most of the New Testament. God used his relationship with Paul at one point and with Mark at another to keep these two men going when either might have failed. Barnabas did wonders with encouragement!

When Paul arrived in Jerusalem for the first time following his conversion, the local Christians were understandably reluctant to welcome him. They thought his story was a trick to capture more Christians. Only Barnabas proved willing to risk his life to meet with Paul and then convince the others that their former enemy was now a vibrant believer in Jesus. We can only wonder what might have happened to Paul without Barnabas.

Barnabas encouraged Mark to go with him and Paul to Antioch. Mark joined them on their first missionary journey but decided during the trip to return home. Later, Barnabas wanted to invite Mark to join them for another journey, but Paul would not agree. As a result, the partners went separate ways, Barnabas with Mark and Paul with Silas. This actually doubled the missionary effort. Barnabas's patient encouragement was confirmed by Mark's eventual effective ministry. Paul and Mark were later reunited in missionary efforts.

Barnabas's story is told in Acts 4:36-37; 9:27–15:39. He is also mentioned in 1 Corinthians 9:6; Galatians 2:1, 9, 13; and Colossians 4:10.

The Race

We can be like Barnabas. And we can encourage people by simply affirming them for a character trait (discipline, loyalty, integrity, honor, and so forth), for making progress in a specific area, or for a job well done (similar to race spectators shouting out, "Looking good!"). We can encourage by coming alongside and running with them, listening, comforting, and meeting a need. And we can encourage by reminding them of God's promises—what Paul did for the Thessalonian believers:

> We tell you this directly from the Lord: We who are still living when the Lord returns will not meet him ahead of those who have died. For the Lord himself will come down from heaven with a commanding shout, with the voice of the archangel, and with the trumpet call of God. First, the Christians who have died will rise from their graves. Then, together with them, we who are still alive and remain on the earth will be caught up in the clouds to meet the Lord in the air. Then we will be with the Lord forever. So encourage each other with these words. (1 THESSALONIANS 4:15-18)

This message of hope should encourage us no matter what we are going through.

The Result

Stop and think about people you can encourage—with a comment, a note, a call, a pat on the back, a reminder of the hope and joy found in Christ. This loving act begins with sensitivity, seeing people as individuals who need a word from God through you. That's everyone, certainly, even those who look so self-assured, successful, and carefree—we *all* harbor secret fears, misgivings, and hurts, and we all need comfort and encouragement.

Be a Barnabas.

My Story

```
The crowd is silent. The runners are lined up, waiting.
Bang! The gun goes off, and another race starts. As a part
of the high school cross-country team for the last three
years, I have grown used to this.
```

I start to pick up speed, digging my spikes in the grass and lifting up with every step. By the half-mile mark, I am breathing hard, wondering why I choose to put myself through this year after year.

As I pass a runner from another team, I breathe out a quick "good job," which she returns.

At that moment, a bond is made. An acknowledgment that we are both struggling and working toward the same goal: finishing. Even though we are from different teams and are racing against one another, we share something in common. There in that field, all of a sudden, every runner becomes a fellow teammate, all working themselves to their limits, all in need of support and encouragement.

The same can be said of our walk with God. It is not an easy race to run, and it is by no means short. But there are other runners, all striving to finish the race well, with whom we can find a common ground in recognizing God's love for us. The Christian journey can be grueling, but it does not have to be embarked on alone. We can count on others to support us when we feel like we can't take another step, and we can also carry their burdens when they need it. It is only with the help that God provides through our fellow brothers and sisters that we can "run with endurance the race God has set before us" (Hebrews 12:1).

Boyi

Think It Through

1. In running, who have you encouraged through your words or your example? How have you encouraged another runner in a race?
2. Who is the most positive, encouraging person you know? What's his or her secret?
3. Reflecting on your relatives, friends, people at church, coworkers, and neighbors, who do you think definitely needs comfort or encouragement?
4. Today, what will you do to comfort or encourage at least two of those people?

On Running

How often should I eat?

Whether dieting or not, *do not skip meals*. Your performance will drop in as little as six hours without eating. Grazing is a good option, especially for endurance athletes, but make sure you are grazing on good foods and aren't eating a lot of excess calories. Also, avoiding a coffee-and-donut breakfast and opting for something more nutritional will help you to manage your eating. A sugar-laden, empty-calorie breakfast can be hypoglycemic, decreasing your blood sugar levels and leaving you wanting more to eat.

JOURNAL

_____

_____

_____

_____

_____

RUNNING LOG

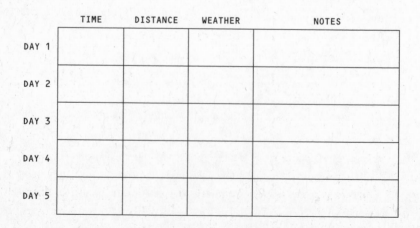

	TIME	DISTANCE	WEATHER	NOTES
DAY 1				
DAY 2				
DAY 3				
DAY 4				
DAY 5				

GIVE ENCOURAGEMENT

Although most runners run alone or with one running partner, many affiliate with a running club or organization, often participating with members in a race to raise money for a ministry or charity. Besides giving and receiving encouragement and holding each other accountable for putting in the miles, members gain the satisfaction of working together to reach a higher goal.

Accountability, encouragement, working together—actually, that sounds like church. And speaking of church, here's what the writer of Hebrews had to say about believers encouraging each other:

> *Let us hold tightly without wavering to the hope we affirm, for God can be trusted to keep his promise. Let us think of ways to motivate one another to acts of love and good works. And let us not neglect our meeting together, as some people do, but encourage one another, especially now that the day of his return is drawing near.* (HEBREWS 10:23-25)

Christians should meet regularly for corporate worship, teaching, service, fellowship, and as this passage highlights, motivating and

encouraging each other, especially because the finish line is close—
"the day of [Christ's] return is drawing near."

The Runner

Oh, hi . . . what was the question? What church do I attend? Uh . . .
CCC—that's Central Community Congregation. You know, the big
one downtown on Main Street.

How often do I attend? Well, I try to get there as often as possible.
Of course, Christmas and Easter are a must—wouldn't miss those services for anything. The music is incredible. And then . . . actually, I'd
love to go more often . . . and I used to go every week, and not just
Sunday mornings; we had a great small-group Bible study. But I got
so busy at work, with trips and all. And now with the kids and their
traveling teams (almost all the events conflict with church), we spend
most of the weekend driving, and I bring my laptop to get stuff done
during the breaks. On those free weekends, we welcome the break and
sort of veg out at home.

Now I'm feeling guilty. I haven't been in a while, and they (I mean
"we") have a new pastor, and he's quite the preacher. I heard a sermon
online and was impressed and even learned something. I suppose we
should get back in the habit, but so much is going on . . . I don't know
what to give up.

The Race

These days, worship services and other church gatherings often
get bumped by work responsibilities, social events, concerts, sports
(races?), and other activities. We can easily take church for granted and
not realize the value of "meeting together." What a mistake!

The Hebrews passage begins with hope that is based upon God's
promises. Then the writer adds an intriguing line: "Let us think of ways
to motivate one another to acts of love and good works." In other words,
even though we know God and what he says in his Word, we need to

be reminded and motivated . . . and encouraged. The clear implication is that when we neglect involvement and input from other believers, we may lose hope and stop living the way we should. We need each other.

The Result

Church is not just for receiving; it's a place where we *give*—encouragement, leadership, service, motivation, and accountability. It's where we use our spiritual gifts to glorify God and build up the body of Christ—*his* people in *that* place.

You have a valuable contribution to make. When you "neglect meeting together," you are missed. Make church a priority, and go with the intention of encouraging someone.

My Story

In our couples' small group, we had fun together, studied together, and even set exercise goals together. That may seem strange, but for us it just seemed logical. Our get-togethers would sometimes include "feats of strength" challenges—push-ups, sit-ups, pull-ups, wall sits, and for the more adventurous, handstand push-ups. Not only did we prepare by studying the week before, we also physically conditioned in anticipation of showing off our strength. Yes, we were competitive. We upped the next challenge as some of us decided to run the half marathon, farther than most of us had ever run. Pat, Dan, Jeremy, Alison, and I were on board, and our spouses supported it.

No problem, I thought. *I run two to three times a week for about four miles at a time. I can work up to 13.1 miles, right?* However, my training was sporadic at best. I ran six miles a few weekends before the race and eight miles another weekend with Jeremy in a thunderstorm.

The date arrived, and it was memorable—in a negative way. We had record-setting rain that weekend, and it rained during the whole race. It should have been called the Chicago half "rain and mudathon" because I had to run through a mud pit to get to the starting line. I was drenched, my shoes and legs were muddy, and I didn't anticipate the pain after the race. Oh yeah, and the Band-Aids didn't stick to my chest region very long.

I said I would never run that long of a distance ever again. Little did I know that two years later I would renege on that statement.

I had finished graduate school and completed a year-long project at work, and now I needed a new challenge. I worked out consistently but had never set a significant physical goal in my life. It was time to run the Chicago Marathon on 10-10-10, a memorable date for sure. My wife, Stephanie, didn't take me seriously at first. Eventually she was on board, and I signed up with Team World Vision to raise money to help provide clean water to children in Africa. I had a new group to train with, and we scheduled runs together every Saturday morning starting eighteen weeks prior to the race. Did I mention the runs started at 6:00 a.m.? I'm not a morning person, but we did it to beat the summer heat. We had fun and were determined to train hard. When we gathered after our long training runs and then hobbled off to our cars, I was usually thinking, *This is farther than I have ever run before; our bodies are amazing.*

Family and friends gathered to cheer me on while I ran the marathon. They spread out along the course at twenty different locations. It was great seeing all of them— exactly what I needed despite the smiles I gave that I hoped would mask the pain and fatigue. The run was hard and everything didn't go as planned, but I finished and I'm happy with my performance.

Groups helped enable me to be successful—family, friends, fellow marathon training partners, and Team World Vision all contributed to realizing my goal. Group bonds were formed, memories were created, and goals were achieved together.

Will I do this again? Absolutely!

Steven

Think It Through

1. What running groups are you aware of? What has been your relationship with them?
2. What groups of Christians do you regularly meet with (worship service, Sunday school class, small group, committee or board, etc.)? How have you been encouraged by those meetings and individuals in those groups?
3. What hinders you from becoming more involved in church? Who do you think you could encourage there?
4. What steps will you take to make regular involvement in church a priority for you? What will you do to encourage your brothers and sisters in Christ?

On Running

What should I eat after I run?

You should replace lost carbohydrates right after running—the first two hours are crucial. Sports drinks can be very beneficial. A small amount of protein with your carbohydrates will help more glycogen to form. (Glycogen is the stored energy in your muscles—the body's primary source of energy.) Without a good store of glycogen, your body will not recover well and give you the energy you need for your next workout. Also, within the first four hours you'll want to consume 1.5 grams of carbohydrate per kilogram of body weight so you fully replenish your glycogen.

JOURNAL

_____

_____

_____

_____

_____

RUNNING LOG

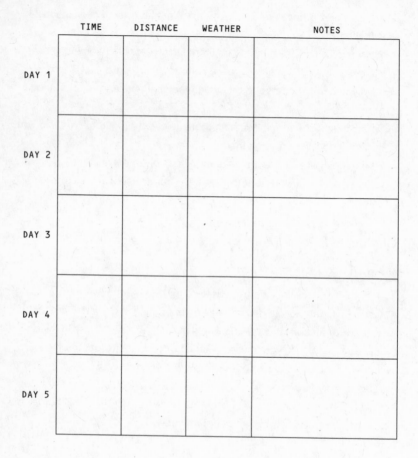

	TIME	DISTANCE	WEATHER	NOTES
DAY 1				
DAY 2				
DAY 3				
DAY 4				
DAY 5				

KEEP PRESSING FORWARD

Almost by definition, a race involves runners pushing their limits, straining to win. So in virtually every race, competitors come to a moment of truth when they must endure and run through their pain, exhaustion, and mental fatigue toward the finish line. Except, perhaps, for world-class and other uniquely gifted runners, just about all who run a marathon experience "hitting the wall," the point where all physical, mental, and emotional resources seem to have been spent and they are running on empty. This occurs at the end of the "serious stage" or in the "encouragement stage" of the race. Runners don't think they can take another step, yet they do . . . and another . . . and another.

A person doesn't have to be a runner to hit the wall. A combination of physical, relational, financial, and emotional setbacks can stop us and make us think we can't go on. Paul and other first-century Christians certainly knew that feeling, and Paul wrote about it. As you read this passage, picture the great apostle as a "coach" urging his runners on:

We now have this light shining in our hearts, but we ourselves are like fragile clay jars containing this great treasure. This makes it clear that our great power is from God, not from ourselves.

We are pressed on every side by troubles, but we are not crushed. We are perplexed, but not driven to despair. We are hunted down, but never abandoned by God. We get knocked down, but we are not destroyed. Through suffering, our bodies continue to share in the death of Jesus so that the life of Jesus may also be seen in our bodies. (2 CORINTHIANS 4:7-10)

We are like "fragile clay jars"—we know this for sure at the "wall." But because we have God's power, we don't depend on our own strength to run and finish. We won't be "crushed," "driven to despair," or "destroyed."

The Runner

He first felt the pain at fifteen miles. It wasn't much then, just a slight stitch in the side. But now it was almost unbearable—under the rib cage, pushing up into the right lung. He had altered his breathing and slowed his pace, but nothing seemed to help. The only thing good about it, he thought, was that he had almost forgotten about his other pains and issues: the constant sting of sweat in his eyes as it ran down across the dried, salty residue on his forehead; the skin rubbed raw even through generous applications of Vaseline; the blisters, formed, broken, and now bleeding.

After the first hour, his muscles ached, throbbing with each step. Now they were numb. Twenty-two miles. *This must be the wall*, he thought. *I'll never make it. I should quit like those others. More than four miles to go.* But he remembered his three months of preparation, his family and friends who had encouraged him, and his goal. And he kept moving.

Suddenly a gust of crosswind threw him off stride. He stumbled a bit but regained form and ran around a corner, to the last water station. Reaching down to the table, he took a cup and, walking slowly, swirled the contents in his mouth and swallowed. He grabbed another cup and poured it over his head, letting the water soak his hair and run down his chest and back. He took another and added its contents to the refreshing rivulets down his neck.

Then joining the other runners, he plunged on. Crunching discarded cups with each painful step, he continued, now almost hobbling toward his goal. Crowds lined the streets and cheered as he passed:

"You can do it!"

"You're almost there!"

"Looking good!"

Their faces blurred, and their voices faded.

Just a mile to go . . . one agonizing step after another, gasping for breath with a mouth of cotton, running on legs of lead with pain in every muscle and joint.

Then he saw it. Penned in large letters, hanging above the street, the word he had longed to see: FINISH. Mustering every ounce of strength, he moved steadily through the last strides of the torturous journey, determined to sprint to the end. Finally, with arms raised in triumph, he crossed the finish line.

The Race

You've been there, struggling through a long run in foul weather (cold rain, humidity, heat) or fighting to finish that 10K, half marathon, or marathon. You know the feelings and the mental games where quitting seems like a good option. So what keeps you going? Probably the knowledge that you trained well, the expectations of family and friends, the sight of the finish line, and most of all, your commitment to your goal.

We've discussed this during other devotional weeks—the early believers in Corinth and the rest of the Roman Empire were facing a tough point in their "marathon." Tired of being persecuted and struggling to stay strong in an increasingly hostile environment, some were weakening, perhaps to the point of giving up and turning away from their faith.

So Paul acknowledged their suffering, reminded them of their *goal* (to display Christ to their world, even through their suffering) and their *power* (from God who was with them), and challenged them to keep running this great race of faith.

The Result

In your personal marathon, you may have hit the wall. The ache may seem more than you can bear, the hurt more than you can handle. Why keep going? Every step is painful.

Look up—see your heavenly Father urging you on and strengthening your steps.

Look around—see the friends and family who are there for you (much like the "crowd of witnesses" in Hebrews 12:1), who love you, who care for you, and who pray for you. They're cheering right now, knowing you can make it. Remember all the training that has brought you this far—the times of answered prayer, the faith and God's strength through the power of the Holy Spirit that has carried you through the tough times before.

And look ahead. The finish line is there, and Jesus is waiting. He is your goal. Keep your eyes on him . . . and keep running.

My Story

In the early-morning hours of September 6, 2009, somewhere on the streets of Batavia, Illinois, I decided I would not run another marathon. On that damp September day, I ran the Foot Mechanics Half Madness half marathon to help decide if I would attempt another fall marathon—this one with an aggressive time goal. I'd trained well and prepared carefully for race day. I was delighted to run

alongside my most loved and trusted running girlfriend.
I was prepared and relaxed. The day held great promise.

But the farther I ran, the more awful I felt.

The damp asphalt roads stretched out endlessly in front
of me. I struggled up even the smallest inclines. A large
middle section of the race was a "false flat," which became
a curse that nearly broke me. Even though I'd completed two
marathons, six half marathons, numerous ten-mile races, and
countless training miles, I had to fight just to keep going.
I kept thinking that more than twenty-five years of running,
good nutrition, and constant dedication to fitness should
have bought me more comfort and ease in my running by that
point. It just wasn't what I thought it should be. I'd done
all the right things . . . why wasn't it easier?

Later reflection revealed just how many races I'd endured
with that mind-set. Somehow I expected that because of all
the "right things" I'd done to prepare, my race effort would
be more, well, effortless. And it wasn't until training for
my fifth marathon that it occurred to me I'd had the wrong
expectation all along. Races are hard. They're *supposed* to
be hard. And marathons are uniquely grueling. Where did I
ever get the idea that race day was an easy, breezy show of
athletic prowess and pride?

Then I thought how I also carry this same idea about
God's blessings. I expect his blessings to be largely
about my personal comfort—an easy life marked by material
and relational success. This expectation is particularly
prevalent when I put in all the "training" of spiritual
disciplines and outward obedience. But such mistaken
expectations blind me to God's true blessings—especially
those found amidst the pain and struggle, not only on
the racecourse but along life's course. I've discovered
that God has a way of planting his goodness and glory
right in the middle of the struggle. And when I trust his
plan despite the uphill course, I am more apt to see the
treasures he's hidden for me inside the challenges.

And so Marathon Day #5 fast approaches. On that day,

I pray that, somewhere along those 26.2 miles—as my head swears, *Never again!* and my body aches to quit—the Holy Spirit will nudge through the discomfort of the moment to whisper the truth again that God is no less present or powerful despite the challenge, and that his reward sits gleaming at the finish line.

Nancy

Think It Through

1. How did you know you had hit the wall in a long run or race? What carried you to the end?
2. When have you been painfully discouraged, perhaps even tempted to quit, to give up on life or at least on the Christian life? What kept you going?
3. Who are your biggest fans on earth, encouraging you to run well?
4. What can you do to rely on God's strength and not your own? What can help you keep focused on Christ?

On Running

Dietary Goals for Performance

NUTRITIONAL GUIDELINES FOR ATHLETES

- 55–60 percent of calories from carbohydrates
- 25–30 percent of calories from fats—one-third from saturated fats
- RDA of vitamins and minerals
- Sufficient calories dependent on training
- Forced fluids
- DO NOT SKIP MEALS. Performance drops in as little as six hours without eating.
- Avoid the coffee-and-donut breakfast. Over time it can be hypoglycemic.
- Endurance athletes should graze.
- Avoid eating 3–4 hours before a run.
- Drink plenty of water and avoid alcohol.

JOURNAL

_____

_____

_____

_____

_____

RUNNING LOG

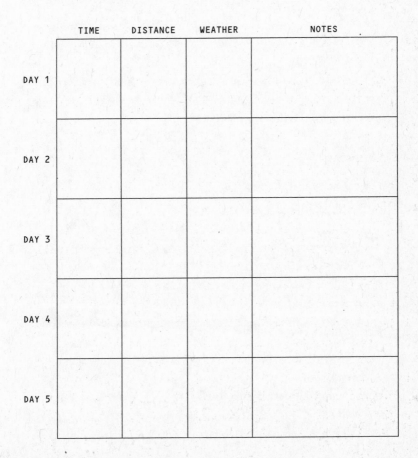

	TIME	DISTANCE	WEATHER	NOTES
DAY 1				
DAY 2				
DAY 3				
DAY 4				
DAY 5				

KEEP PRESSING FORWARD

Most people who run a marathon just want to finish. Certainly they want to do their best, but they have no dreams or delusions about winning the race; for them, finishing is victory enough. That's because they know the difficulty of this task—and for first-time marathoners, the race is probably the longest distance they've ever run. That someone completes a marathon means he or she trained for three months—six days out of every week (with the seventh day for recovery), regardless of weather conditions, potential scheduling conflicts, or other possible excuses for not running. It also means that this runner conquered the "serious stage" of the race and "the wall." Long-distance runners learn discipline, endurance, courage, and faith. They also learn much about themselves and grow in their confidence. In other words, the adversity of the race brought out the best in them.

Beyond running, we have seen that adversity comes in many forms. For most believers in the first century—and so many throughout the world today—the extreme tough times and trials came simply because they were following Christ. But similar to marathon runners, as they endured and pushed through the wall of persecution, they demonstrated the purity of their faith and developed endurance and character. Hear again the powerful witness of Peter and Paul:

> *Through your faith, God is protecting you by his power until you receive this salvation, which is ready to be revealed on the last day for all to see.*
>
> *So be truly glad. There is wonderful joy ahead, even though you have to endure many trials for a little while. These trials will show that your faith is genuine. It is being tested as fire tests and purifies gold—though your faith is far more precious than mere gold. So when your faith remains strong through many trials, it will bring you much praise and glory and honor on the day when Jesus Christ is revealed to the whole world.* (1 PETER 1:5-7)

> *We can rejoice, too, when we run into problems and trials, for we know that they help us develop endurance. And endurance develops strength of character, and character strengthens our confident hope of salvation. And this hope will not lead to disappointment. For we know how dearly God loves us, because he has given us the Holy Spirit to fill our hearts with his love.* (ROMANS 5:3-5)

The Runner

Annie Johnson Flint (1866–1932) lost both parents before she was six years old. She was adopted by a loving couple, but as a teenager, she developed severe arthritis and soon became unable to walk. She had wanted to be a composer and concert pianist, but after her illness made playing the piano impossible, she began writing poetry, setting some of the poems to music. Later in life, she couldn't even open her hands, but she still wrote her poems on the typewriter, typing with her knuckles. One of her best-known poem-songs is "He Giveth More Grace," based on the Bible promises found in James 4:6, Isaiah 40:29, and Jude 1:2.

He giveth more grace as our burdens grow greater,
He sendeth more strength as our labors increase;
To added afflictions He addeth His mercy,
To multiplied trials He multiplies peace.

(Chorus)
His love has no limits, His grace has no measure,
His power no boundary known unto men;
For out of His infinite riches in Jesus
He giveth, and giveth, and giveth again.

When we have exhausted our store of endurance,
When our strength has failed ere the day is half done,
When we reach the end of our hoarded resources
Our Father's full giving is only begun.

(Chorus)

The Race

God wants us to depend totally on him. Centuries ago, through his prophet, the Lord proclaimed to Zerubbabel, "It is not by force nor by strength, but by my Spirit" (Zechariah 4:6), and we've already read Philippians 4:13: "I can do everything through Christ, who gives me strength." Our natural inclination is to try to depend on our own mental and physical power and call on God only in emergencies. But he wants to empower us moment by moment, and that means we must depend on him. Some people learn this lesson only through extreme adversity when their faith is tested and purified. They reach the end of their resources and have no option but to depend on God. And they do . . . and press on to the finish.

The Result

Here's a tough assignment: Thank God for your adversity, your trials. He has promised that they will last only "a little while" (especially in light of eternity) and that they will purify you and form you into the kind of person he can use . . . to his glory.

My Story

I never liked running. I did it because I had to for sports. Put me in a game, and I would run nonstop and go forever; but ask me to run a couple of miles, and I would roll my eyes and pout all the way to the finish line. Now I love to run. What was the change?

Just before college orientation, I participated in an eighteen-day hiking and backpacking trip for incoming freshman. Leading up to the trip, we were told that if we could easily run two miles, we would be prepared for the hike. No problem.

During the trip, we did a variety of activities— canoeing, rock climbing, hiking along Lake Superior, forty-eight hours of solitude—but the trip ended with a ten-mile run back to camp. For someone who ran only when sports required it, this was a long distance. Plus, I hadn't run in the previous two weeks—wouldn't I be out of shape?

We put on our running shoes (what a relief to get out of hiking boots!), tied our laces, and took off. This wasn't a typical road race. We ran around trees, over rocks, and through marshes, and before I even knew it, I had reached the halfway mark. I had already run five miles and felt great!

But around mile seven, I started to drag. Everyone had spread out, so I was pretty much running alone and feeling really tired. At that moment, right when I needed it, a girl I had met only briefly ran up to me and in her sweet Southern voice said, "Dana, you can do it! You're doing great! 'For I can do all things through Christ who gives me strength.'" Then she continued running.

Tears came to my eyes, and I knew I could finish. I had

just hiked for over two weeks with only what I could carry on my back, and God had been with me through it all. He would help me finish. Crossing that finish line, cheered on by the others who had already finished, was one of the greatest feelings in my life. I did something I never thought I could do. And I know that when I needed it most, God had sent Katherine along my path to encourage me with words and Scripture—and I finished strong. I finished that run and have been a runner ever since. Her words not only encouraged me in that moment, but they developed a love of running in me.

I learned that God sees us, hears us, and brings along what we need most, right when we need it.

Dana

Think It Through

1. Why do you admire someone who has completed a marathon? What have you learned about yourself during running adversity?
2. When are you tempted to live on your own strength and not rely on God? Why do you think you are tempted then?
3. In what ways have your "problems and trials" developed your endurance, character, hope, and confidence?
4. What can you do to remind yourself to rely on God's strength at *all* times, not just during adversity?

On Running

Seven Principles of Exercise—Part One

1. THE PRINCIPLE OF INDIVIDUALITY:
All people are created differently. Heredity determines how quickly and to what degree your body adapts to a training program. Any training program must take into account the specific needs and abilities of the individuals for whom it is designed.

2. THE PRINCIPLE OF SPECIFICITY:

Your training program should focus on the areas you specifically want to develop (e.g., breath capacity, leg strength, stride), which will allow you to achieve your training goal (e.g., pace, endurance).

3. THE PRINCIPLE OF DISUSE:

If you stop training, your state of fitness will drop to a level that meets only the demands of daily use.

JOURNAL

_____

_____

_____

_____

_____

RUNNING LOG

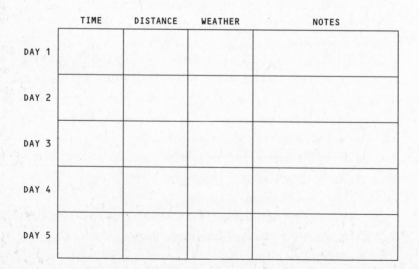

	TIME	DISTANCE	WEATHER	NOTES
DAY 1				
DAY 2				
DAY 3				
DAY 4				
DAY 5				

FINISH STRONG

During any long-distance run, especially when we feel exhausted and in pain, one of the most important decisions we can make is to look forward, to think of what lies ahead—the finish. For some, that means winning a prize or achieving a personal record. For others, the prospect of seeing loved ones waiting for them and cheering them on is all they need. And for all, finishing well is a great achievement.

Seeing the finish isn't easy when we're miles away, in the personal fog of discouragement and doubt. When spectators are trying to encourage us by shouting, "Just a 10K more!" we think, *Six miles to go? How can I possibly run six more miles!* At the aid stations, we pour water on ourselves to somehow cool off; then we try to run again, limping down the course, and wonder how we can ever make it to the end. But we press on, the finish line drawing closer with each painful step.

Knowing that we *have* a finish and knowing what awaits us there should motivate us to run well and finish strong—in the race and in life. That certainly was Paul's attitude:

I don't mean to say that I have already achieved these things or that I have already reached perfection. But I press on to possess that perfection for which Christ Jesus first possessed me. No, dear brothers and sisters, I have not achieved it, but I focus on this one thing: Forgetting the past and looking forward to what lies ahead, I press on to reach the end of the race and receive the heavenly prize for which God, through Christ Jesus, is calling us.
(PHILIPPIANS 3:12-14)

Did you hear those verbs, those decision points? "Forget," "look forward," and "press on"—the past is behind us, over, done, forgiven. The end of the race lies ahead, and with it God's heavenly prize.

The Runner

Florence Chadwick was a marathoner, but in swimming, not running. Born in San Diego on November 9, 1918, she began swimming competitively at the age of ten and competed in her first rough-water swim at eleven.

Florence is remembered for swimming across the English Channel from France to England in thirteen hours and twenty minutes, breaking the record. That was in 1950. A year later, she swam the Channel again, this time from England to France, setting another record at sixteen hours and twenty-two minutes.

In 1952, Florence became the first woman to attempt a twenty-six-mile swim from Catalina Island to the California coastline. About fifteen hours into the swim, as a thick fog settled over the ocean, Florence became disoriented and began to think she would not be able to finish her quest. After swimming for another hour, with the coastline still shrouded in fog, Florence asked to be pulled from the water. It was only after she was in the boat that she learned she was only a mile short of her destination.

Two months later, Florence tried again. The thick fog rolled in again, but this time she kept swimming and reached her goal. She said she made it because she kept a mental image of the finish—the shoreline—as she swam.

The Race

"Seeing the finish," even in her mind, gave Florence the strength to keep going and to finish strong.

In another passage, Paul elaborates on how the present race can feel and what awaits us at the finish, what we can envision:

> We know that all creation has been groaning as in the pains of childbirth right up to the present time. And we believers also groan, even though we have the Holy Spirit within us as a foretaste of future glory, for we long for our bodies to be released from sin and suffering. We, too, wait with eager hope for the day when God will give us our full rights as his adopted children, including the new bodies he has promised us. We were given this hope when we were saved. (If we already have something, we don't need to hope for it. But if we look forward to something we don't yet have, we must wait patiently and confidently.)
> (ROMANS 8:22-25)

We can identify with the "groaning" part. But we can also hope, knowing that a glorious future awaits us in new bodies that will never tire, reunited with our loved ones in the presence of our Lord and Savior.

The Result

Every day the finish line of life gets closer. Knowing that your race will soon end and that rest, reunions, and rejoicing await you should encourage and motivate you now, on every step of your race.

My Story

Miles two and three passed like a stroll through Grant
Park. I didn't even realize when I passed the seven-mile
marker. At mile fifteen I smiled and waved at the cheering
crowd. Nineteen, twenty, twenty-one. They all passed
without much effort.

The crowds thinned after the drink station at the
twenty-third mile, and I no longer had to fight to stay
next to Tammy, my running partner.

All of a sudden, taking another step took focus. Focus
on the goal and not focus on the unshakable desire to just
stop. Stop running and walk.

When I gave in to that nagging voice telling me
everything would feel better if I could just walk a few
steps, I discovered the trick. A few walking steps didn't
satisfy that voice. Once my shuffling run became a walk,
the voice in my head changed its mind and decided walking
wasn't enough; my body actually needed to just stop and
lie down. I longed for that rest, even considered it for a
few minutes, until the authority in Tammy's voice cleared
the mental fog lulling me to follow the soothing voice
that would keep me from finishing my marathon goal.

Between breaths she sang about lifting up my eyes to
the hills because God is where my strength comes from.
I could feel determination set into my face again because
I knew I couldn't let my friend down either. With the
gentle announcement that she was taking requests for the
next song, my mental energy shifted from the ache in my
weary legs to lyrics that might keep my energy moving
forward to the finish line.

Less than an hour later, we bowed our heads to receive
medals placed around our necks. As we gave each other
high fives and hugged despite sticky, salty bodies, I
thanked God for returning my focus to him and the prize
of finishing the race strong.

Angie

Think It Through

1. What experiences of a long-distance race do you tend to forget? Which ones do you think you will always remember? What makes the difference?
2. Which parts of your past do you need to release and forget?
3. Which aspects of God's finish line do you look forward to most?
4. What will you need in order to finish strong?

On Running

Seven Principles of Exercise—Part Two

4. THE PRINCIPLE OF PROGRESSIVE OVERLOAD:
In order to continue improvement, you need to increase the difficulty of your workouts slowly so as not to plateau.

5. THE PRINCIPLE OF HARD/EASY:
On a day following a high-intensity workout, you might need an easy day of training.

6. THE PRINCIPLE OF PERIODIZATION:
This is the gradual cycling of the areas you want to develop (specificity), how hard you train (intensity), and how much you train (volume) to achieve peak levels of fitness for competition.

7. THE PRINCIPLE OF OVERTRAINING:
Overtraining is a condition in which an athlete's adaptive mechanisms are stressed to the point of failure.

JOURNAL

_____

_____

_____

_____

_____

RUNNING LOG

	TIME	DISTANCE	WEATHER	NOTES
DAY 1				
DAY 2				
DAY 3				
DAY 4				
DAY 5				

FINISH STRONG

Every runner knows the feeling of seeing the finish line. Whether the run was five miles through the neighborhood, a 10K, or a marathon, the sight of the finish motivates us to push, to "sprint," to finish strong. And that's true regardless of how we are feeling. Runners tell how they were spent physically and emotionally and ready to quit, and others describe the terrible pain in lungs and legs, but they persevered and felt buoyed by the sight of the finish. Some push so hard at the end that they are wrapped in foil and taken directly to the medical tents. Most cross the line with hands raised in triumph!

The *real* finish is when life ends. As we have noted several times, for most people life is like a marathon, not a sprint—a long-distance run with several stages. Yet unlike a marathon, which ends after 26.2 miles, we don't know the exact location of life's finish line. We do know, however, that our life race is actually pretty short, no matter how long we live; we'll get to that line sooner than many of us expect.

Paul knew his race was nearly over; his finish line was in sight. So he wrote:

*As for me, my life has already been poured out as an offering to
God. The time of my death is near. I have fought the good fight,
I have finished the race, and I have remained faithful. And now
the prize awaits me—the crown of righteousness, which the Lord,
the righteous Judge, will give me on the day of his return. And the
prize is not just for me but for all who eagerly look forward to his
appearing.* (2 TIMOTHY 4:6-8)

Paul was sprinting to the end.

The Runner

Born in the small East African country of Eritrea, Meb Keflezighi (one
of ten children in his family) began life as a survivor, not a runner.
Fleeing the brutal war that was tearing apart their country, Meb and
his family eventually emigrated to America. Meb explains:

*We came to the United States with virtually nothing but the
clothes on our backs and the faith that we were in the Land of
Opportunity, where education could be pursued and hard work
would be rewarded. I had no idea that running was even a
sport when we arrived in the States. My running journey began
with a timed mile in my seventh grade phys ed class. I got all
my competitive experience in the United States through middle
school, high school, and college meets.*[1]

Eventually Meb became a world-class long-distance runner, winning
the silver medal in the marathon at the 2004 Athens Olympics. But a
series of injuries followed that triumph. So when Meb entered the New
York City Marathon in 2009, he was determined to win. He recalls:

*Victory . . . would be sweet for a number of reasons. To begin with,
the race hadn't had an American winner since Alberto Salazar won*

. . . *in 1982. Second, I had never had a victory in my previous*
11 marathon starts. . . . Furthermore, many "experts" thought my
career was over, and even I considered retirement in 2008 because of
injury. I also wanted to do something special in honor of my friend
and former training partner, Ryan Shay, who died of cardiac arrest
in 2007 while we were competing in the Olympic trials marathon
in Central Park. Perhaps most important, my parents, wife, and
children were at the race. I envisioned accomplishing something
special with them in attendance.[2]

Meb describes how that marathon ended:

I was expanding the lead running along Central Park South and
heading toward Columbus Circle, where the crowds were thick
and loud. The noise was deafening and pushed me toward the
finish. I heard shouts of "USA! USA!" and "Go Meb!" It was the
thrill of a lifetime. Turning right and back into Central Park,
I had a 34-second lead with 385 yards left.

    I popped my USA singlet a couple of times. I flashed double
thumbs-up and waved to the crowd. I was trying to take in the
moment. I was also thinking, Rein yourself in. Don't celebrate too
much. Get to the finish. I was about to win my first marathon.
I was about to become the first American winner in New York
in 27 years. I had believed all along I could do it. But I couldn't
believe it was actually happening. All those close calls. All
those unlucky breaks and weird injuries. Food poisoning. Stress
fractures. Ruptured quads. All kinds of problems at the wrong
times. The countless hours of rehab and cross-training.

    Then there were all those people who thought I was over the
hill. All those who said I'd never win a major marathon. But this
was more than proving them wrong. This was about getting the
most out of myself, about seeing my Run to Win philosophy in
action. I thanked God for listening to my prayers. . . .

*The tears were welling up. I was overwhelmed with emotion.
. . . I saw [my wife], seven months pregnant, holding Sara and
Fiyori. I saw my mother. We all were crying. My father was there,
the guy who told me I could beat the world at the 2000 Olympics.
I had told him it would take time to do that. It had taken nine
years, but I had finally beaten the world in New York.*[3]

The Race

Meb remembered his goal, heard the cheers, and saw the finish with
his family waiting for him there. So he gave everything he had and
raced to victory.

Sitting alone and chained in the dark and damp Roman prison,
Paul *saw* his finish line, and he, too, was determined to finish well. He
also knew that he would not be the only victor but would join all those
who trust in Christ as their Savior. Paul had given his all; he had run
well; he would wear the victor's crown!

What a marvelous promise! What a courageous race! What an
amazing life of faithful service to the Lord! May the same be said for us.

The Result

You know the finish line is there, whether or not you can see it. No
one drops out of this race; eventually, one way or another, life ends
for everyone. But the meaning of the finish is profoundly different
for those who run for Christ and his Kingdom. Let the knowledge of
who and what awaits you motivate you to run strong and hard and
finish well.

My Story

I don't know if it's just my partial Scottish heritage,
but something in me responded the first time I heard
the quote from Eric Liddell: "When I run, I feel his

pleasure." Those words make running about a lot more than healthy exercise.

I've been running all my life, though I admit most of it has involved chasing a soccer ball. I grew up in South America, and much of my childhood was filled with the kind of daily, energetic activities that make you wonder as an adult, *How did I do all that stuff?*

I didn't try formal running until we returned to the U.S. when I was in seventh grade. The track team in my junior high school was a no-cut team, so the coach had to find an event for everybody who showed up. For him, the 440 was a good way to separate the runners from the boys. Those who didn't show specific promise in some other event found themselves assigned to run the 440. One time around the track . . . too far to sprint all the way, not nearly far enough to expect a water stop on the back straightaway. What I remember are 440 races that looked to me like the start of the Boston Marathon. Four or five serious runners on the starting line with a multitude of wannabes bunched close behind. Two moments in each of those races are indelibly recorded for me.

The first mental picture comes as I lean into the first turn and look ahead at an unbroken single-file wall of runners hugging the inside line around the entire turn. Something was beautiful about all those bodies daring gravity together to cut the corner as close as possible. Sometimes I laughed in the sheer joy of the moment. This perspective, of course, reminds me that I was among the last runners.

Somewhere during the back straight section, a predictable separation would take place. The pack became two packs. By the time my group was starting into the second curve, the lead runners were sprinting for the finish line. By then a gap of forty or fifty yards would have opened between the contenders and the rest of us. When we came out of the turn, it was a whole new race. No one was in front of us.

We in the back were as serious about finishing as any of the others who were already in the showers. And this is when the second indelible image flashes on my mental screen, this one with sound. The crowd often responded to our efforts by cheering us in. And we responded to their encouragement by battling it out across the finish line, stepping on the tape that was already growing a little mold. Those moments have always caused me to marvel over the joy of finishing. Of course winning is fun, but winning is the refined form of finishing. Unless you finish, you can't win.

As my life has reached that phase where physical output has more to do with good memories than present exploits, I find it comforting to know that the writer in the Bible who gave us such great word pictures of exertion in describing the Christian life saved a special one when he saw the tape approaching: "I have fought the good fight, I have finished the race, and I have remained faithful" (2 Timothy 4:7). I, too, have had my share of wins along the way, but in the end what I want to do is finish, and finish well. The longer I live, the more I understand that when I run, I feel his pleasure.

Neil

Think It Through

1. In what ways has the sight of the finish to a long run or race affected how you ran? What award awaited you when you finished?

2. Although most people have no idea how long they will live, where do you think you are in life's race—at what stage of the marathon?

3. Paul said he had "fought the good fight"—what did that mean for him? What does the "good fight" look like for you?

4. What did Paul's statement that he had "remained faithful" say about him? What does "remaining faithful" mean for you? In what ways does the finish line and what awaits you affect how you live?

On Running

Tapering

Just before a very important race you should back off a little from your training—"taper." This will allow time for all the damaged micro-constructions of muscle to reach full repair. It also will allow for carbohydrate replenishing and to increase and prepare your mental and psychological state. You shouldn't back off on intensity, just on distance. Long-distance runners shouldn't taper more than a week. You face the risk of detraining (getting out of shape) if you taper for too long.

JOURNAL

RUNNING LOG

	TIME	DISTANCE	WEATHER	NOTES
DAY 1				
DAY 2				
DAY 3				
DAY 4				
DAY 5				

"MY STORY"
CONTRIBUTORS

Many thanks to the following runners who shared their running stories with us:

- Brian Barton
- Becky Brandvik
- Todd Busteed
- Tiffany Chang
- Kara Conrad
- Mike Cox
- Sarah Drake
- Amy Duren
- Kim Freking
- Joshua Grubb
- Steven M. Heerdt
- David Hubbard
- Elizabeth Hubbard
- Mark Jackson
- Leanne Lacewell
- Frank Lee
- Dana Niesluchowski
- Mary Pappas
- Rich Peachey
- Don Parrish
- Angie Reedy
- Don Rice
- Nancy Rice
- Kaitlyn Rustemeyer
- Matthew Schulte
- Michael Smith
- Cheryl Steplight
- Katy Swanson
- Jermaine Taylor
- Anthony Trendl
- Ellen VandeLune
- Dave Veerman
- Tony Vuksinic
- Becky Williams
- Neil Wilson
- Christy Wong
- Caroline Yasuda
- Boyi Zhang

SCRIPTURE INDEX

5K RACE TRAINING PLAN

WEEK	MON	TUE	WED	THU	FRI	SAT	SUN
1	Rest	10 min. walk 10 min. run 10 min. walk	10 min. walk 15 min. run 10 min. walk	Rest	10 min. walk 1 mile run 10 min. walk	2 x 10 min. run with 2 min. recovery walks	Rest
2	4 x 5 min. run with 1 min. recovery walks	10 min. walk 10 min. run 5 min. walk 10 min. run	30–45 min. walk	2 x 1 mile run with 2 min. recovery walks	Rest	2 x 10 min. run with 1 min. recovery walks	Rest
3	4 x 5 min. run with 1 min. recovery walks	5 min. walk 10 min. run 2 min. walk 10 min. run	30–45 min. walk	2 x 1 mile run with 2 min. recovery walks	Rest	2 x 15 min. run with 2 min. recovery walks	Rest
4	5 min. walk 1 mile run 2 min. walk 1 mile run	2 x 15 min. run with 2 min. recovery walks	30–45 min. walk	2 x 1 mile run with 2 min. recovery walks	Rest	3 x 10 min. run with 1 min. recovery walks	Rest
5	5 min. walk 2 mile run 5 min. walk	Cross-train	5 min. walk 2 mile run 5 min. walk	Rest	45 min. speed walk	3 x 10 min. run with 1 min. recovery walks	Rest
6	2 miles	Cross-train	2 x 15 min. run with 2 min. recovery walks	Rest	2 miles	3 miles	Rest
7	2 miles	Cross-train	3 x 15 min. run with 2 min. recovery walks	Rest	2 miles	4 miles	Rest
8	3 miles	Cross-train	3 miles	Rest	2 miles	4 miles	Rest
9	2 miles	Cross-train	3 miles	Rest	2 miles	2 miles	Rest
10	3 miles	Rest	2 x 10 min. run with 1 min. recovery walks	Easy 30 min. walk	2 miles	Rest	RACE!

10K RACE TRAINING PLAN

WEEK	MON	TUE	WED	THU	FRI	SAT	SUN
1	Rest	10 min. walk 10 min. run 10 min. walk	10 min. walk 15 min. run 10 min. walk	Rest	10 min. walk 1 mile run 10 min. walk	2 x 15 min. run with 2 min. recovery walks	Rest
2	3 x 10 min. run with 2 min. recovery walks	5 min. walk 10 min. run 2 min. walk 10 min. run	30-45 min. walk	2 x 1 mile run with 2 min. recovery walks	Rest	3 x 1 mile with 1 min. breaks	Rest
3	3 x 10 min. run with 2 min. recovery walks	5 min. walk 10 min. run 2 min. walk 10 min. run	30-45 min. walk	2 x 1 mile run with 2 min. recovery walks	Rest	3 x 1 mile with 1 min. breaks	Rest
4	5 min. walk 2 mile run 5 min. walk	3 x 15 min. run with 2 min. recovery walks	30-45 min. walk	3 x 1 mile run with 2 min. recovery walks	Rest	4 miles with 1 min. walk break every 25 mins.	Rest
5	3 miles	Rest	5 min. walk 2 mile run 5 min. walk	Rest	3 miles	4 miles with 1 min. walk break every 25 mins.	Rest
6	3 miles	Rest	3 miles	Rest	3 miles	4 miles (no break)	Rest
7	3 miles	Rest	4 miles	Rest	3 miles	5 miles	Rest
8	3 miles	Rest	4 miles	Rest	3 miles	6 miles	Rest
9	4 miles	Rest	5 miles	Rest	3 miles	6 miles	Rest
10	3 miles	Rest	5 miles	Rest	3 miles	4 miles	Rest
11	3 miles	Rest	4 miles	Rest	3 miles	3 miles	Rest
12	2 miles	Rest	3 miles	Easy 30 min. walk	2 miles	Rest	RACE!

BEGINNERS' HALF MARATHON TRAINING PLAN

WEEK	MON	TUE	WED	THU	FRI	SAT	SUN
1	Rest	10 min. walk 10 min. run 10 min. walk	10 min. walk 15 min. run 10 min. walk	Rest	10 min. walk 1 mile run 10 min. walk	2 x 15 min. run with 2 min. recovery walks	Rest
2	3 x 10 min. run with 2 min. recovery walks	5 min. walk 10 min. run 2 min. walk 10 min. run	30–45 min. walk	2 x 1 mile run with 2 min. recovery walks	Rest	3 x 1 mile with 1 min. breaks	Rest
3	5 min. walk 2 mile run 5 min. walk	3 x 15 min. run with 2 min. recovery walks	30–45 min. walk	3 x 1 mile with 2 min. recovery walks	Rest	4 miles with 1 min. walk break every 25 mins.	Rest
4	3 miles	Rest	3 miles	Rest	3 miles	4 miles	Rest
5	3 miles	Rest	4 miles	Rest	3 miles	5 miles	Rest
6	3 miles	Rest	5 miles	Rest	3 miles	8 miles	Rest
7	3 miles	Rest	5 miles	Rest	3 miles	10 miles	Rest
8	4 miles	Rest	5 miles	Rest	4 miles	11 miles	Rest
9	4 miles	Rest	6 miles	Rest	4 miles	12 miles	Rest
10	4 miles	Rest	5 miles	Rest	4 miles	9 miles	Rest
11	3 miles	Rest	4 miles	Rest	4 miles	8 miles	Rest
12	3 miles	Rest	4 miles	Easy 30 min. walk	2 miles	Rest	RACE!

EXPERIENCED
RUNNERS' HALF MARATHON TRAINING PLAN

WEEK	MON	TUE	WED	THU	FRI	SAT	SUN
1	Rest	3 miles	3 miles	3 miles	Rest	6 miles	Cross-train
2	Rest	3 miles	3 miles	3 miles	Rest	7 miles	Cross-train
3	Rest	3 miles	4 miles	3 miles	Rest	5 miles	Cross-train
4	Rest	3 miles	4 miles	3 miles	Rest	9 miles	Cross-train
5	Rest	3 miles	5 miles	3 miles	Rest	10 miles	Cross-train
6	Rest	3 miles	5 miles	3 miles	Rest	7 miles	Cross-train
7	Rest	3 miles	6 miles	3 miles	Rest	12 miles	Cross-train
8	Rest	3 miles	6 miles	3 miles	Rest	13 miles	Cross-train
9	Rest	3 miles	7 miles	4 miles	Rest	10 miles	Cross-train
10	Rest	3 miles	7 miles	4 miles	Rest	15 miles	Cross-train
11	Rest	4 miles	6 miles	3 miles	Rest	8 miles	Cross-train
12	Rest	3 miles	4 miles	2 miles	Rest	Rest	RACE!

BEGINNERS' MARATHON TRAINING PLAN

WEEK	MON	TUE	WED	THU	FRI	SAT	SUN
1	Rest	4 miles	3 miles	1 hour run	Rest	6 miles	Cross-train
2	Rest	4 miles	3 miles	1 hour run	Rest	7 miles	Cross-train
3	Rest	4 miles	4 miles	3 miles	Rest	9 miles	Cross-train
4	Rest	4 miles	3 miles	6 miles	Rest	10 miles	Cross-train
5	Rest	4 miles	5 miles	4 miles	Rest	7 miles	Cross-train
6	Rest	5 miles	7 miles	3 miles	Rest	12 miles	Cross-train
7	Rest	5 miles	7 miles	3 miles	Rest	13 miles	Cross-train
8	Rest	5 miles	8 miles	4 miles	Rest	10 miles	Cross-train
9	Rest	5 miles	8 miles	4 miles	Rest	15 miles	Cross-train
10	Rest	5 miles	8 miles	4 miles	Rest	16 miles	Cross-train
11	Rest	5 miles	9 miles	4 miles	Rest	12 miles	Cross-train
12	Rest	5 miles	9 miles	4 miles	Rest	18 miles	Cross-train
13	Rest	5 miles	10 miles	5 miles	Rest	20 miles	Cross-train
14	Rest	5 miles	8 miles	4 miles	Rest	12 miles	Cross-train
15	Rest	4 miles	6 miles	3 miles	Rest	8 miles	Cross-train
16	Rest	3 miles	Rest	3 mile jog	Rest	2 mile jog	Marathon

NOTES

1. Meb Keflezighi with Dick Patrick, *Run to Overcome* (Carol Stream, Illinois: Tyndale House Publishers, 2010), 3.
2. Ibid., 3–4.
3. Ibid., 209–210.

DISCOVER THE REAL MEANING OF VICTORY WITH NEW YORK CITY MARATHON WINNER MEB KEFLEZIGHI

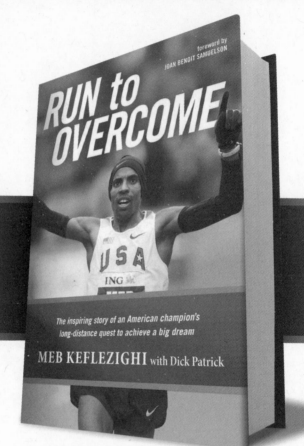

What happens when your dreams come crashing down? Faced with this question, one runner fought to overcome a career-threatening injury, personal loss, and a future that had never looked more uncertain—without losing faith in God or himself. *Run to Overcome* is the inspiring true story of an Eritrean refugee who became an American champion. Join Meb Keflezighi on his long-distance quest to run and win—and learn how he defeated the odds to win the 2009 New York City Marathon.